Basic Cardiac Rhythms: The Visual Nurse's Guide

Tyler C. Scanlon, MS, BSN, RN

Registered Nurse, Cardiac Stress Lab

Guest Lecturer, Applied Exercise Physiology

NOTICE

The criteria presented here are based upon a consensus of previously published information in addition to the author's own experiences and viewpoints. Readers should seek additional references regarding ECG interpretation to continually improve their skills. While topics presented may include causes and treatments where appropriate, the primary focus of this text will include the proper identification of selected cardiac rhythms. Readers should review package inserts and user manuals for any medications, therapeutic agents, or devices as directed by the USFDA. The author, editor, and publisher disclaim responsibility for adverse effects resulting from omissions and undetected errors or adverse results obtained from the use of the information in this book. Application of the information in any situation remains the professional responsibility of the licensed individual performing such interventions. Information presented in this text is not medical advice and it is the responsibility of the reader to verify accuracy of all materials presented.

Finally, I chose to write this book in a laid back and conversational style. I've written for academia and peer review in the past and find I *prefer* to write as if we're in the same room together. Let's keep it loose here.

Thanks for picking up a copy!

If you're reading this, chances are your current or future role involves rapid cardiac rhythm interpretation. This can be one of the most challenging topics for students to learn. Of course, I am partially biased in that this text is presented from the nurse's perspective however, it is my hope that this text will provide great benefit to nursing students, new nurses, cardiac monitor technicians, paramedic students, and medical students alike!

My goal is to provide you with the most amount of information in as few words possible (hence the graphics). They say a picture is worth a thousand words. If you wanted to read for the sake of reading you would have picked up a copy of War and Peace by Leo Tolstoy.

My hope is that you can use the pictures presented as a quick reference if you need a topic refresher once you complete the reading. For this reason, each topic is presented in the following format:

1. **What is it?**
2. **What does this mean?**
3. **Why should we care?**

TAKE HOME POINTS:

✓ **These are presented after each topic. Think of them as a, "What do I need to know about this topic if I only have 10 seconds to review this page?" type of review.**

As you read, take special care to appreciate the underlying *concept* for each rhythm strip instead of just memorizing waveform appearances. This will help to make sense of *why* the waveforms appear the way that they do. Remember that each rhythm strip tells a *story* of what's happening behind the scenes (at the micro and macro cellular level). We're simply observing a 30,000-foot view of what's occurring beneath our electrodes.

For my wife, Cortney, and our daughter, Charlie.

Table of Contents

INTRODUCTION

ELECTROCARDIOGRAM (ECG)

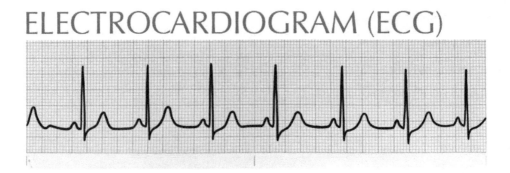

What is an electrocardiogram?

Assuming an average heart rate of 70 beats per minute, the heart will beat over 100,000 times per day. This translates to over 2.8 *billion* beats over the course of an average lifespan. Will the first heartbeat that you experience resemble your last? How would we know?

The heart contains two macro-systems which we'll review: plumbing and electrical. One moves blood volume. The other stimulates the muscle to perform the work of moving this volume.

Aside from taking the heart out of the chest (not recommended), how can we visualize its activity? Echocardiography, cardiac magnetic resonance (MRI), and other modalities afford visualization of the structural and contractile properties of the heart but fail to provide direct information related to conduction.

How would we know if a person were predisposed to conduction abnormalities or lethal arrhythmias? How would we know if anti-arrhythmic medications are working effectively? If your patient had been experiencing dizziness, palpitations, or loss of consciousness recently, how would you know if it were related to fluid volume status, a weakened pump (heart), or cardiac rhythm abnormalities (or a combination of all)? What if we had a tool that provided macro-level information related to chemical activity on the cellular level which allowed us to detect minor abnormalities prior to them becoming problematic?

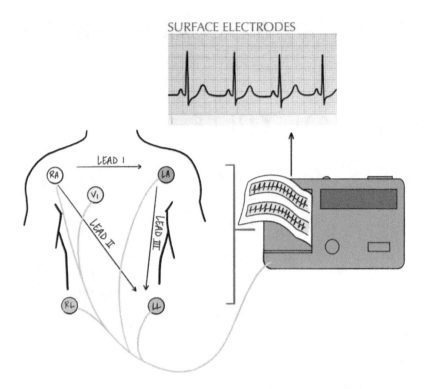

An electrocardiogram (ECG) is an electrical rendition that tells the story of the physical events occurring in the heart with each beat (electro = electrical, cardio = pertaining to the heart, gram = record or picture). Surface electrodes are placed on the skin at specific anatomical positions that provide a recording of activity below the surface.

What does this mean?

The ECG is a diagnostic tool, useful for detecting abnormal conditions. These abnormal conditions include conduction abnormalities and arrhythmias. Arrhythmia (or dysrhythmia) is the term used to describe abnormal cardiac conductions and their importance is largely related to the effect they have on total cardiac output, with a few exceptions.

Why should we care?

Electrocardiograms help guide treatment for both emergent events and chronic conditions. Longitudinal changes may be the result of genetic predispositions, medication therapies, structural changes, tissue death, conduction delays of electrical origin, and more[1]. Before we learn how to read an ECG, let's review a few basic principles as they pertain to cardiac arrhythmias.

TAKE HOME POINTS:

- ✓ An electrocardiogram (ECG) is an electrical rendition of the physical events occurring in the heart
- ✓ The ECG is a diagnostic tool, useful for detecting abnormal conditions including arrhythmias
- ✓ Arrhythmia, or sometimes *dys*rhythmia is the term used to describe abnormal cardiac rhythms and their importance is directly related to their effect on total cardiac output

CHAPTER 1: BASIC CARDIAC PHYSIOLOGY

CARDIAC OUTPUT INFLUENCE

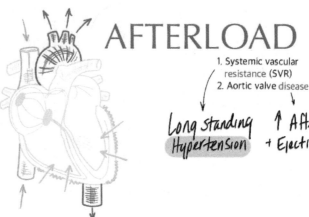

AFTERLOAD

1. Systemic vascular resistance (SVR)
2. Aortic valve disease

Long standing
Hypertension

↑ Afterload
+ Ejection Pressures

PRELOAD

1. Venous return
2. End diastolic volume
3. Circulating blood volume
4. Respiratory pump
5. Skeletal muscle pump

Inspiration decreases
Intrapleural pressures
to "pull" blood back

CONTRACTILITY

1. End diastolic influence
   (Frank-Starling law)
2. Sympathetic nervous
   system stimulation
3. O2 supply

→ ↑ Stretch
= Stronger rebound

Hormones
Neurotransmitters
Medication

Mild hypoxemia
stimulates
contractility increases

Epi/Norepinephrine
Thyroid
Dopamine

How does blood flow through the heart?

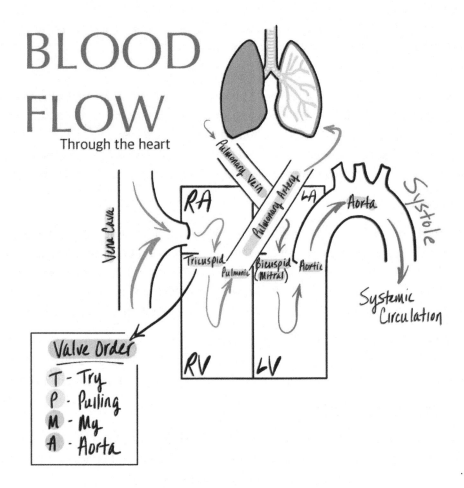

To build a structure that will house our cardiac rhythm knowledge, we first need to lay a concrete foundation. Reviewing basic anatomy and hemodynamic principles followed by review of the cardiac conduction system will provide this foundation.

How does blood flow through the heart?

Like the homes in which we live, the heart has two major systems: electrical and plumbing. Am I the first person to present this groundbreaking analogy? No. But can I relay it more simply than it previously has been? That's my hope. The electrical system (the cardiac pacemaker cells) is responsible for generating the impulse that signals the cardiac *muscle* to contract, sending blood forward. The two systems depend upon one another, and you cannot have one without the other. What does this mean?

What does this mean?

Think about this: living cells need oxygen to survive. This includes cardiac pacemaker cells. Our pacemaker cells are *fed* primarily by the epicardial coronary arteries that lie on top of the heart. The right coronary artery (RCA) for example, feeds the *right* side of the heart in addition to other territories[2].

If something were to disrupt that flow, say a large coronary plaque or blockage, this would starve the right side, inferior portion, and likely posterior portions of the heart.

Now, which specialized pacemaker cells lie within the right (atrium) side of the heart? That's right, the Sino-atrial (SA) node, and the SA node sets the pace for the rest of the heart under normal conditions. For this reason, the SA node is referred to as the "pacemaker of the heart". If we starve the SA node it gets sick. If it gets sick, it becomes weaker.

This is one reason patients that have experienced heart attacks involving the RCA might develop profound bradycardias (brady = slow, cardia = heart) and/or heart blocks[3]. The RCA feeds the SA node in 55% of individuals, along with the AV node and bundle of His in 90%[4]. So... if the heart cannot beat strongly enough to move blood forward and to also to feed itself, *electrical* activity may *also* slow. If electrical activity slows dramatically, then so does blood flow. Herein lies the problem.

Why should we care?

The next question is, "Which came first, the chicken or the egg?" It depends. A heart attack itself is an event with potential to progress to irreversible ischemia, cellular compromise, cardiac arrest, and sudden death. This is estimated to account for as much as 80% of sudden cardiac deaths in Western countries[5]. What ultimately results in death, however, is the electrical arrest stemming from irritable and oxygen starved heart cells. So, which came first? You'll be happy to hear, it still depends.

Individuals might also have faulty conduction (think ion channels) and/or repolarization issues, causing dysrhythmias, sometimes lethal ones. Others *acquire* this because of blockages leading to cardiac oxygen deprivation. An oxygen hungry heart is an irritable heart and if tissue dies, it's gone.

The previous graphic depicts blood flow through the heart[6].

Deoxygenated blood enters the right side of the heart through the vena cava → then travels into the right atrium→ through the tricuspid valve and into the right ventricle and finally → through the pulmonary artery toward the lungs. Following oxygenation in the lungs:

The blood travels back to the left side of the heart through the pulmonary vein → then into the left atrium → through the bicuspid (mitral) valve and into the left ventricle → then sent through the aorta and into systemic circulation.

"Try Pulling My Aorta" is the mnemonic I use to remember the order of the valves blood passes through as it progresses through the heart (tricuspid, pulmonic, mitral, aorta). Another great one is to "Tri it before you Bi it" (Tri = tricuspid first on the right; Bicuspid/mitral; on the left). Everything mentioned relates to total cardiac output which we'll discuss next.

TAKE HOME POINTS

- ✓ The two major systems of the heart are the electrical and plumbing systems
- ✓ The electrical system initiates blood movement and oxygen delivery which feeds itself via the coronary arteries
- ✓ If the electrical system fails, blood flow slows
- ✓ If the plumbing system is blocked, blood flow slows
- ✓ Failure of one system directly affects the performance of the other

How do we measure the output of the heart?

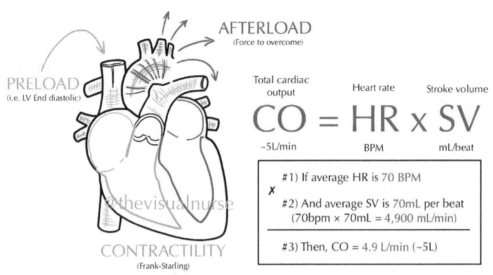

CARDIAC OUTPUT

AFTERLOAD
(Force to overcome)

PRELOAD
(i.e. LV End diastolic)

CONTRACTILITY
(Frank-Starling)

@thevisualnurse

Total cardiac output ~5L/min

Heart rate BPM

Stroke volume mL/beat

$$CO = HR \times SV$$

#1) If average HR is 70 BPM

#2) And average SV is 70mL per beat
(70bpm × 70mL = 4,900 mL/min)

#3) Then, CO = 4.9 L/min (~5L)

What is cardiac output?

Cardiac output (CO) by its simplest definition is the output of the heart (although the entire cardiovascular system should be considered). The term tells you exactly what it is. What it fails to provide is a unit of time associated with the output (kind of important!). Why is this important?

Cardiac output is the total output of the heart each *minute*. The amount of blood moved with a *single* stroke (or beat) of the heart is called the *stroke* volume (SV). If only there were a way to relate this to the overall output each minute... If we know the volume of each stroke, and the rate of the heart (HR)... What if we multiply to find the stroke volume per minute[7] (CO = HR x SV)? Bingo. I guess the term *"stroke volume per minute"* doesn't exactly roll off the tongue so instead, we use the term cardiac output.

What does this mean?

There are certain factors that may increase or decrease heart rate and stroke volume, resulting in overall changes to total output per minute (CO). These are listed on the next page.

CARDIAC OUTPUT INFLUENCE

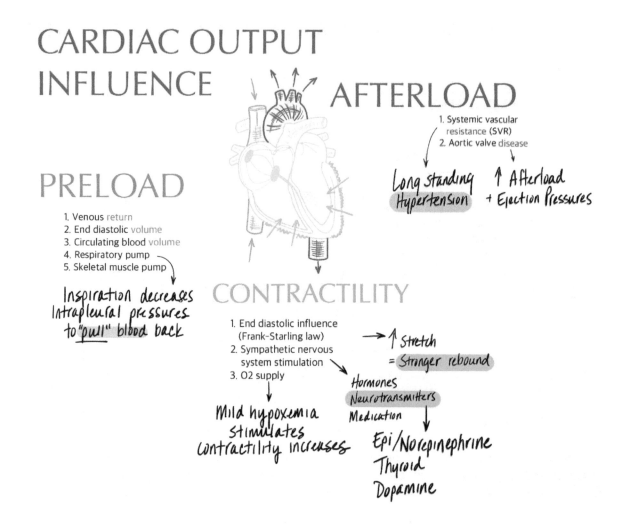

AFTERLOAD

1. Systemic vascular resistance (SVR)
2. Aortic valve disease

Long standing Hypertension

↑ Afterload + Ejection Pressures

PRELOAD

1. Venous return
2. End diastolic volume
3. Circulating blood volume
4. Respiratory pump
5. Skeletal muscle pump

Inspiration decreases Intrapleural pressures to "pull" blood back

CONTRACTILITY

1. End diastolic influence (Frank-Starling law)
2. Sympathetic nervous system stimulation
3. O2 supply

↑ Stretch
= Stronger rebound

Hormones
Neurotransmitters
Medication

Mild hypoxemia stimulates Contractility increases

Epi/Norepinephrine
Thyroid
Dopamine

Preload: Preload is the degree of myocardial stretch prior to contraction and is influenced in part by the amount of blood present in the chambers of the heart prior to expulsion[8]. Like a rubber band, the greater the stretch, the stronger the recoil (to a finite degree). Preload influences the Frank-Starling mechanism in this way. It is largely represented by the left ventricular end diastolic volume[9] (during the filling phase) and is influenced by venous blood return to the heart.

Venous return is greatly influenced by total circulating blood volume (in addition to other factors). In cases of blood loss for example, venous return might expectedly decrease. During periods of activity and exercise preload is increased in part, due to the skeletal muscle pump and the respiratory pump[7]. Skeletal muscles throughout the body squeeze blood back to the heart through one-way valves located in our veins when these muscles contract.

The respiratory pump functions to "pull" blood back to the heart due to pressure gradient increases[7]. In the pleural cavity during inspiration, negative pressure is produced when the diaphragm flattens and contracts, which increases venous return. Blood wants to flow from areas of high pressure to low pressure.

Afterload: Afterload is the resistance the heart must overcome to eject blood into circulation. Hypertension (including pulmonary) forces the heart to work harder. Additionally, valvular diseases like aortic valve stenosis narrow the pathway for blood to leave the heart. Replacing a stenotic aortic valve or reversing hypertension decreases the afterload (resistance) the heart must overcome. This puts less strain on the heart to deliver the same amount of volume per beat (stroke volume) thereby increasing cardiac output assuming all other factors remain constant[8].

Contractility: The strength of the squeeze. Factors are listed in the image above[9]. During the fight or flight response for example, circulating catecholamines (like epinephrine and norepinephrine) increase which stimulates a more frequent and forceful contraction.

Comparatively, medications called beta blockers function to block adrenergic receptors to decrease rate and strength of contraction, which produces an overall decrease in blood pressure in addition to other effects.

Why should we care?

These factors above influence either heart rate or stroke volume, both of which have a direct effect on overall cardiac output. Remember, CO (L/min) = HR x SV.

TAKE HOME POINTS

- ✓ Cardiac output is the total output of the heart each *minute*
- ✓ Factors that may increase or decrease heart rate and stroke volume resulting in overall changes to total output include preload, afterload, and contractility

Impairments in cardiac output

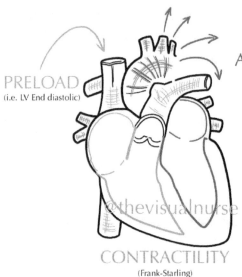

CARDIAC OUTPUT
(HR X SV)

PRELOAD
(i.e. LV End diastolic)

AFTERLOAD
(Force to overcome)

Signs of impaired cardiac output
- Hypotension
- Chest pain
- Weak peripheral pulses
- Hypoxia
- Cardiac dysrhythmias
- Palpitations
- Dyspnea, Fatigue, Dizziness
- Decreased urine output
- Cool, clammy skin

@thevisualnurse

CONTRACTILITY
(Frank-Starling)

What is impaired cardiac output?

Impaired cardiac output = decreased blood flow = decreased oxygen delivery. That's the idea behind all of this.

What does this mean?

If the heart is moving less blood, we should expect to feel the symptoms of impaired oxygen delivery. The following may be present:

Hypotension: This may be due to low circulatory volume, a weakened pump, impaired vascular tone, or a combination of these, in addition to others.

Chest pain: For example, "demand angina" is the term used to describe chest pain due to oxygen demands exceeding supply[10]. Cool, clammy skin may accompany this as we attempt to shunt blood to the heart and body's core to feed the most vital organs.

Weak pulses: What is true for hypotension and poor perfusion is also true here. Weak and thready pulses may accompany.

Hypoxia: Decreases in blood volume and concentration results in decreased hemoglobin delivery, potentially leading to decreases in oxygen delivery. In severe cases, this may result in increased anaerobic metabolism causing increased acid production, leading to acidotic states[7].

Cardiac dysrhythmias: Cardiac tissue that's deprived of oxygen may become an irritable tissue. Irritable tissue may act out and produce extra or erratic beats[11,12]. This may manifest as palpitations, syncope, or death depending upon the severity of the cause.

Dyspnea, fatigue, dizziness: May be attributed to decreased oxygen delivery. Acute agitation may also be one of the first signs of acute hypoxemia and hypoxia.

Why should we care?

Sustained abnormal cardiac conductions may poorly affect cardiac output. For this reason, the manifestations above warrant mention as we progress through basic rhythm interpretation.

TAKE HOME POINTS

- ✓ Impaired cardiac output -> decreased blood flow -> decreased oxygen delivery
- ✓ Sustained abnormal cardiac conductions may poorly affect total cardiac output

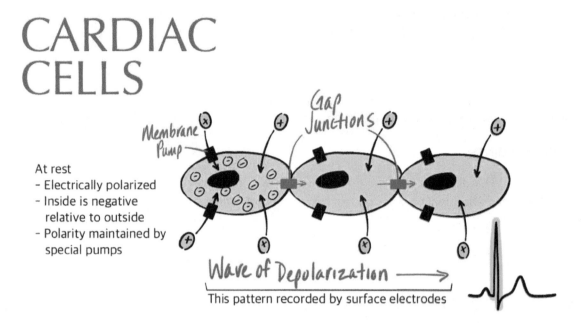

At rest
- Electrically polarized
- Inside is negative relative to outside
- Polarity maintained by special pumps

What are cardiac cells?

Cardiac pacemaker cells are unlike any other. They possess automaticity, meaning they require no outside stimulus to initiate an action potential. The heart will beat on its own for a period if removed from the body due to this. In addition to the property of automaticity, they're excitable and conductive. This means that neighboring cardiac cells can react to stimuli and can pass that stimulus to the next cell in line. These are the functions of the cardiac pacemaker cells: to initiate the impulse and excite neighboring cells.

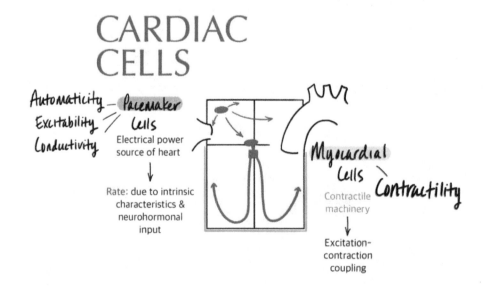

Myocardial cells by comparison are primarily used for their contractile purposes, although these cells may generate an impulse under particular circumstances[11]. The pacemaker cells of the SA node possess the greatest intrinsic rate and ability to spontaneously depolarize, preventing others from having to do so… in a perfect world. The cells of the SA node happen to depolarize more frequently than downstream sites including the AV junction and purkinje fibers, one reason sinus rhythm predominates at a rate of 60-100 beats per minute[11] (BPM).

At rest, cardiac cells maintain a negative inner charge relative to their environment and when these cells depolarize, the net charge becomes more positive by the influx of ions. As this occurs, an activation wavefront of positive potentials is produced and sensed by the surface ECG electrodes as an *upward positive* deflection as this wavefront travels *toward* the positive electrodes[13].

What does this mean?

As this wave of depolarization occurs, the impulse is passed from cell to cell by specialized "doorways" called gap junctions that allow for rapid ion sharing, communication, and impulse transmission. Interestingly, gap junctions will also close off to protect neighboring cells when intracellular ion levels increase during myocardial infarction as a protective mechanism[14].

After depolarizing, specialized membrane pumps move the ions back to their resting states, and the cells are ready for the next wave. The goal with this process is to pass the signal to the myocardial cells, which stimulates contraction, which produces cardiac output, which allows organ perfusion, and life to continue. Whew.

Why should we care?

This pattern of depolarization and repolarization is captured by the surface (on the skin) electrodes and produces the P-Q-R-S-T deflections that we refer to as a cardiac rhythm. It's just a biologically artistic rendition of what's occurring at the cellular level but due to this, we can determine when something or multiple things are out of balance.

An overview of differences between pacemaker cells and myocardial (myo = muscle, cardia = heart) cells is presented in the next section.

TAKE HOME POINTS

- ✓ Cardiac cells are excitable and conductive
- ✓ The pattern of depolarization and repolarization is captured by the surface (on the skin) electrodes and produces the P-Q-R-S-T deflections
- ✓ These deflections describe what's occurring at the cellular level, indicating when something or multiple things are out of balance

CONDUCTION PATHWAY

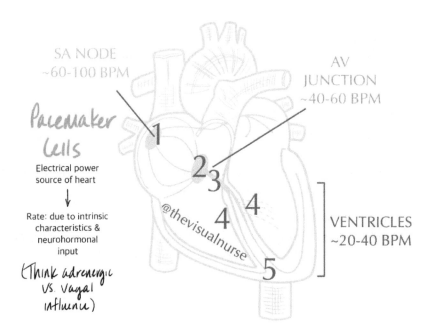

SA NODE
~60-100 BPM

AV
JUNCTION
~40-60 BPM

Pacemaker
Cells

Electrical power
source of heart

↓

Rate: due to intrinsic
characteristics &
neurohormonal
input

(Think adrenergic
vs. vagal
influence)

@thevisualnurse

1

2 3

4 4

4

5

VENTRICLES
~20-40 BPM

What is the cardiac conduction pathway?

Electricity and plumbing. These are the two macro-systems working synchronously within the heart. We've covered blood flow through the heart, and now we turn to the conduction pathway: the path an impulse follows through the heart to tell the heart *muscle* when to beat. I like to think of this conduction pathway as a high-speed train travelling along the tracks from top to bottom. This will make sense when we talk about ventricular rhythms later.

Think of the electrical impulse as the brains behind the operation and the cardiac muscle as just that, the muscle. All brawn and no brain, only contracting when they're told to do so by the specialized pacemaker cells (exceptions exist).

What does this mean?

Pacemaker cells: the electrical power source of the heart. Inherent rates differ among these special cells based upon location (sinus, junctional, or ventricular/purkinje system) and can be influenced by neuro-hormonal input. Think adrenergic stimulation versus vagal stimulation. Beta adrenergic receptor stimulation increases *chronotropy* (speed of contraction; chrono = time), *inotropy* (strength of contraction; ino = I know my own strength), *dromotropy* (conduction velocity) and lusitropy (cardiac relaxation time; lus = loose = faster relaxation for filling)[9]. Beta adrenergic receptors in the heart elicit this response when stimulated by catecholamines. Beta *blocking* medications work to lessen this effect and decrease blood pressure as a result.

Vagal nerve stimulation increases gastro-intestinal motility but has the opposite effect on the heart when stimulated[15]. For this reason, "bearing-down" or performing a vagal maneuver is sometimes used to terminate supraventricular tachycardias (SVT), or to help differentiate certain arrhythmias from one another by slowing the heart rate.

The pacemaker cells of the SA node are greatly innervated by the sympathetic and parasympathetic nervous systems[6] and typically set the heart rate between *60 - 100 times per minute*. If they fail, have an impulse blocked, or die, the AV junction is next in line at *40 - 60 BPM inherently*, followed by ventricular cells at *20 - 40 BPM*[16,17]. With each progression down the line, we run the risk of decreased cardiac output partly due to a decrease in heart rate. Remember, cardiac output = HR x SV.

Shown in the image above, the natural pathway of cardiac conduction should look like this:

1. The impulse begins with the SA node setting the pace
2. From here the impulse travels along the inter-nodal pathways shown between 1 & 2 above, to the AV junction. *There is a slight delay here which is the reason the P-R segment is flat on the ECG.* This pause allows for complete ventricular filling. (As a side note: this is one danger of sustained rapid heart rates. Without the pause to fill, the ventricles eject less blood resulting in decreases in cardiac output)
3. From the AV node, we head to the bundle of His followed by
4. The left and right bundle branches, finally giving way to
5. The purkinje fibers, located near the terminal parts of the ventricles at the apex

Because the ventricles are thick and slow to conduct relative to the rest of the heart, the impulse speeds up *quite a bit* in the purkinje fibers allowing for complete and simultaneous ventricular contraction[13]. The result is maximum blood expulsion from the ventricles.

Why should we care?

Thankfully the back-up sites listed above exist if the SA node were to fail. These sites may keep us beating long enough to have an artificial pacemaker put in or other treatment performed to keep things ticking along if needed. Now that we understand the *normal pathway* of a cardiac impulse let's look at how this affects the upward and downward deflections on the cardiac rhythm strip in the next section.

TAKE HOME POINTS

- ✓ Think of the electrical impulse as the brains behind the operation and the cardiac muscle as just that, the muscle
- ✓ Myocardial cells are the machinery performing the work of contraction resulting in systole
- ✓ Pacemaker cells set the rate of contraction
- ✓ Rates are typically between 60 – 100 BPM, 40 – 60 BPM, and 20 – 40 BPM for sinus, junctional, and ventricular sites, respectively
- ✓ Normal cardiac conduction begins with the SA node and terminates in the purkinje fibers

ECG RATES
REFERENCE SHEET

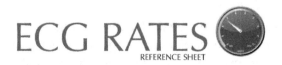

SINUS:		JUNCTIONAL:		VENTRICULAR:	
BRADYCARDIA	<60	BRADYCARDIA	<40		
INTRINSIC	60-100	INTRINSIC	40-60	INTRINSIC	20-40
TACHYCARDIA	>100	ACCELERATED	60-100	ACCELERATED	~50-100
		TACHYCARDIA	100-150	TACHYCARDIA	>100
		SVT	>150		

SA NODE
~60-100 BPM

AV
JUNCTION
~40-60 BPM

VENTRICLES
~20-40 BPM

@thevisualnurse
www.thevisualnurse.com

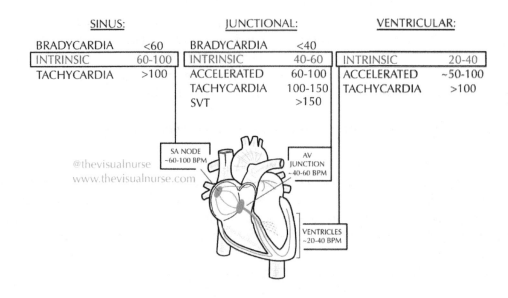

CHAPTER 2: HOW DO WE RECORD ELECTRICAL ACTIVITY?

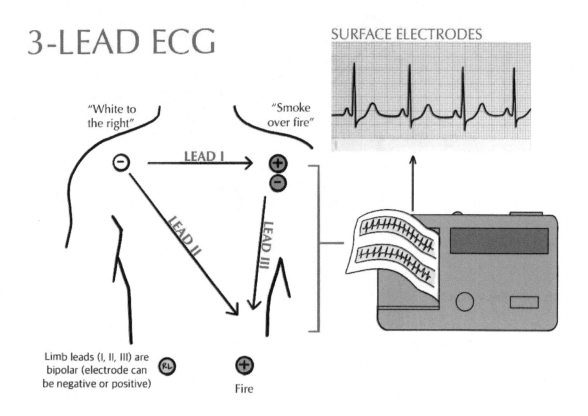

Cardiac vectors

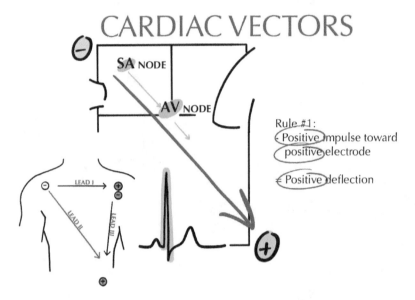

What is a cardiac vector?

The heart is located just behind and to the left of the sternum. The cardiac vector describes the direction in which the wave of depolarization travels through the heart[1] (the flow of electricity). Rule #1 of interpreting basic cardiac rhythms is understanding that an impulse traveling *toward a positive* electrode will produce a *positive (upward) deflection*. If the impulse is traveling *away* from a positive electrode a *negative (downward)* deflection is produced[1]. This is a major foundation of understanding basic cardiac rhythms.

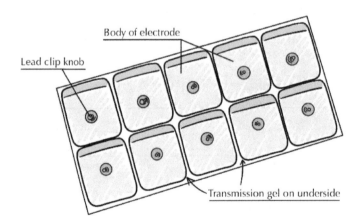

Electrodes sense electrical activity and transmit to leads and acquisition modules (next page).

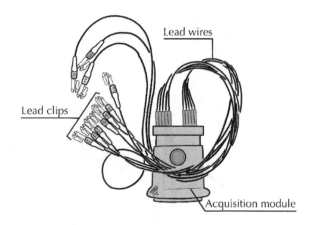

Acquisition modules house leads that provide a graphical representation of electricity sensed by electrodes.

What does this mean?

The natural progression of depolarization in a normal healthy heart is downward and to the left from the SA node to the ventricles. We'll discuss limb leads in the upcoming sections but for now understand that *Lead II* typically follows the most natural path of depolarization in the (healthy) heart and for this reason is preferred by many as the primary "rhythm strip" or "rhythm lead". Of course, other leads are useful for differentiating arrhythmias but are beyond the scope of our discussion at present.

Previously, we discussed the way that cardiac cells depolarize. We mentioned that they are relatively negative at rest and when they depolarize, they're becoming more positively charged. When this is initiated at the SA node, a wave of depolarization occurs from top to bottom. As this positive wave travels toward our electrode, it produces a positive deflection on our ECG. Conversely, an impulse traveling away from this electrode should produce a negative deflection. Turn to Chapter 1 for a refresher on cardiac cell depolarization.

Why should we care?

We're beginning to tie together the concepts of what happens on the cellular level and how these changes manifest in the form of deflections that ultimately form our rhythm strip. Making this connection will serve as the basis for all your cardiac rhythm expertise! Next, we'll discuss standard lead placement and begin to look at the segments of the cardiac cycle and it's deflections, the PQRS & T.

ECG GRAPH PAPER

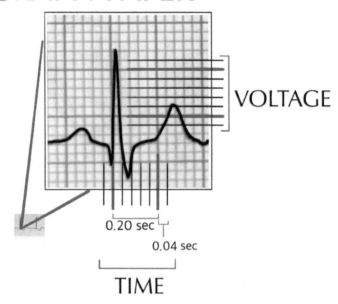

Of course, we need a standardized method of documenting and comparing rhythms. Our ECG graph paper allows us to do this. Special paper measuring voltage along the horizontal lines and time along the vertical lines allows for precise measurement and description of cardiac waveforms. We'll discuss this in greater detail in the coming sections.

TAKE HOME POINTS

- ✓ Rule #1 of interpreting basic cardiac rhythms is understanding that a *positive* impulse traveling *toward a positive* electrode will produce a *positive (upward) deflection*
- ✓ If the impulse is traveling *away* from a positive electrode, a *negative (downward)* deflection is produced
- ✓ The heart depolarizes downward and to the left
- ✓ *Lead II* follows the most natural path of depolarization in the heart

Leads: what are they reading?

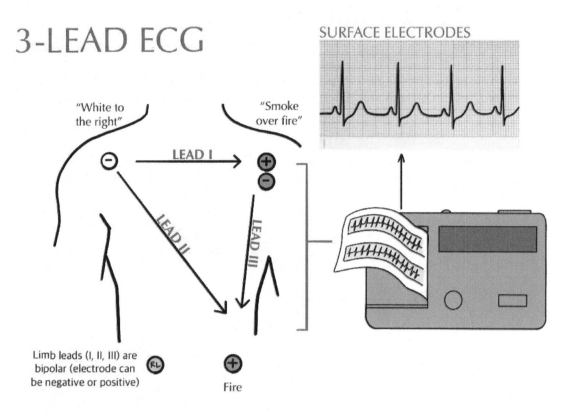

What are limb leads?

Limb leads derive their name from the placement of the associated electrodes... on the limbs of the patient. For the 12-lead ECG, limb electrodes are placed distal to the shoulders and hips[1] although these are usually modified to the upper chest and left and right lower quadrants for continuous 3 and 5 lead telemetry monitoring in the hospital setting, as above. Think white to the right, smoke over fire, clouds over grass. Leads are reading electrical activity that's transmitted between two separate electrodes (above).

What does this mean?

The "white to the right" trick was how I remembered proper lead placement when putting patients on telemetry monitoring as a student since the corresponding module leads are color coordinated by position (this may vary by location and manufacturer). I still sometimes catch myself thinking it to double check my placement. The image above shows a standard 3-lead placement, and the next image shows the 5-lead set-up. Again, these are named so because the electrodes are placed on the limbs of the patient: the right and left arms and legs.

These electrodes are bipolar, meaning the electrode can be negative or positive. In fact, leads I and III have the left arm (LA; black) electrode in common. The difference is this electrode is positive for lead I and negative for lead III. Remember, the heart depolarizes downward and to the *LEFT*. Therefore, we expect to see *positive* deflections in lead I in a normal healthy heart[13].

In lead III, the black left arm electrode is the negative electrode and the left leg (LA; red electrode) is the positive electrode. What does this mean? The heart depolarizes *DOWNWARD* and to the left. This means that the left leg (red) electrode would be the positive electrode receiving the impulse from the heart and should also produce mostly *positive* deflections with some exception.

Why should we care?

We can see why lead II is often preferred as the "rhythm strip" or primary "rhythm lead". It follows the most natural progression of depolarization through the heart (down and to the left). Here's the 5-lead set-up:

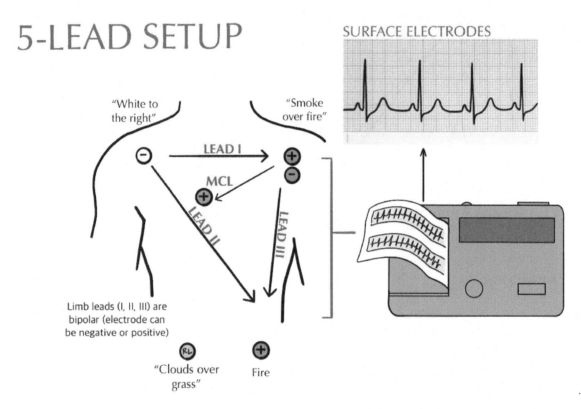

The addition of a 5th electrode (MCL; the modified chest lead), typically corresponding with the V1 position of the 12-lead ECG allows for additional views[17]. Lead II and V1 are my two favorite leads to use for rhythm monitoring if available, since they're extremely useful for P wave investigation (Note the V1 electrode sits almost directly over the right atrium). The MCL (or V) electrode is brown when we set up telemetry. I like to tell myself that the heart loves chocolate, to remember the position.

TAKE HOME POINTS

- ✓ "White to the right, smoke over fire, clouds over grass, the heart loves chocolate"
- ✓ Limb leads are named so because the electrodes are placed on the limbs of the patient
- ✓ They're bipolar, meaning the electrode can be negative or positive

CHAPTER 3: THE CARDIAC CYCLE

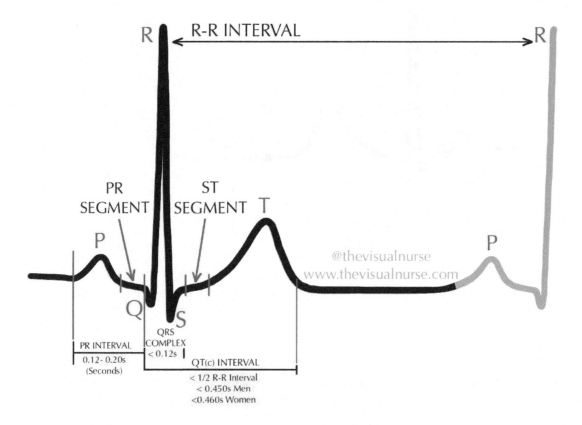

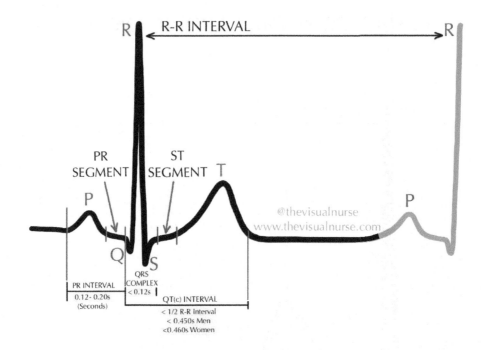

"So when are we actually going to get to rhythm strip interpretation?" If this describes what you're thinking at this point, then here we go.

What is the cardiac cycle?

The graphic above provides an overview of the cardiac cycle, a fancy term that describes the events composing a single heartbeat. This includes the preparation for the next beat, or cycle.

What does this mean?

Each wave and segment has a name and event with which it is associated. Every event in the cycle also has a normal range and each occurs within fractions of a second. What's important to understand is that each cardiac cycle *should* produce a pulse. For example, if you palpate a radial pulse on your patient, you should feel a rebound for each R wave in the cycle. If a cardiac cycle occurs and a pulse is not felt, that beat may not have perfused adequately. We want to ensure electrical matches mechanical.

This is often easy to identify when taking a manual blood pressure. If a patient has frequent premature ventricular contractions (introduced in Chapter 8) you will often hear a pause with each PVC on auscultation. The stroke volume associated with PVCs may be insufficient to produce a palpable pulse[18] and this is also a danger associated with ventricular tachycardia.

Why should we care?

Each measurement and segment play an important role in cardiac rhythm interpretation. To recognize what is abnormal we must know what the normal cycle looks like first, in textbook form.
From these intervals, we can then build upon this foundation and cover the most common (and some uncommon) telemetry rhythms that you'll come across. Rhythm interpretation is one of the most

challenging topics for new nurses, paramedics, and medical residents, but it doesn't have to be! Next, let's look at each component of the cardiac cycle.

TAKE HOME POINTS

- ✓ The cardiac cycle represents a single heartbeat
- ✓ Each cardiac cycle should produce a pulse
- ✓ If a cardiac cycle occurs and a pulse is not felt, that beat may or may not have perfused adequately

The P wave

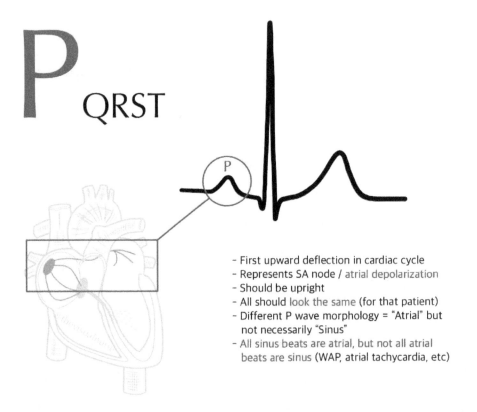

- First upward deflection in cardiac cycle
- Represents SA node / atrial depolarization
- Should be upright
- All should look the same (for that patient)
- Different P wave morphology = "Atrial" but not necessarily "Sinus"
- All sinus beats are atrial, but not all atrial beats are sinus (WAP, atrial tachycardia, etc)

We've covered positive deflections on the ECG and what they actually mean. Now let's dig into the cardiac cycle and begin by examining the first positive deflection, the P wave.

What is a P wave?

First to the party: the P wave. The P wave is the first positive deflection in the cardiac cycle (PQRST) and represents _atrial_ depolarization[13]. Interestingly, the _SA node_ depolarizes *before* the P wave appears, but the event is too small to be seen on the surface ECG. Instead, it's commonly taught that the P wave represents SA node AND atrial depolarization for this reason[19].

The single most important lesson to impart here is that the P wave represents atrial depolarization, and the QRS complex represents ventricular depolarization. This is important because the SA node is what we refer to as the "pacemaker" of the heart. It quite literally sets the pace for the timing of each cardiac cycle[11] resulting in atrial and ventricular depolarization.

What does this mean?

P waves should be upright in leads I and II, and they should all look the same (for a specific patient anyway). My P waves may look different than yours, and yours may look different than your neighbor's. What's important is that your P waves all look the same and that they arrive 60 to 100 times per minute. If a P wave appears that looks different than the rest, we refer to it as an *atrial ectopic* beat. Ectopic simply means *from an abnormal origin*. If an atrial beat comes early, we call it a premature atrial contraction (PAC). Premature atrial contractions are common in the general population and are typically benign but may be felt as occasional palpitations[20].

What do we mean by sinus or atrial? Think of it this way: all sinus beats (P waves) are atrial, but not all atrial beats are sinus. Why? Because the SA (sinus node) is located *within* the right atria. Case in point: the "wandering atrial pacemaker" rhythm strip shown below. This has nothing to with hardware or cardiac devices (i.e. implantable cardiac pacemakers). Instead, this rhythm refers to multiple atrial sites competing with one another to take the lead on setting the pace for the cardiac cycle. As a result, we see multiple P wave morphologies that appear different from one another.

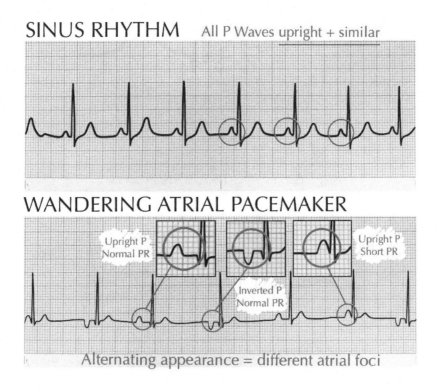

Why should we care?

In the case of the wandering atrial pacemaker, the patient has multiple atrial foci that are depolarizing[17]. P waves do not look the same because they're taking a different route to the AV junction. In this case, we can't name the rhythm as sinus. Instead, we call it a wandering atrial pacemaker, because the pacemaker of the heart is "wandering" throughout the atria (not really, but it describes the absence of a true, set sinus pacemaker). We'll look more closely at these rhythms later. For now, understand that the P wave represents SA node and/or atrial depolarization and sets the pace for the rest of the heart.

TAKE HOME POINTS

- ✓ The P wave is the first positive deflection in the cardiac cycle and represent atrial depolarization
- ✓ The SA node is referred to as the pacemaker of the heart
- ✓ All sinus beats are atrial but not all atrial beats are sinus

The PR interval and PR segment

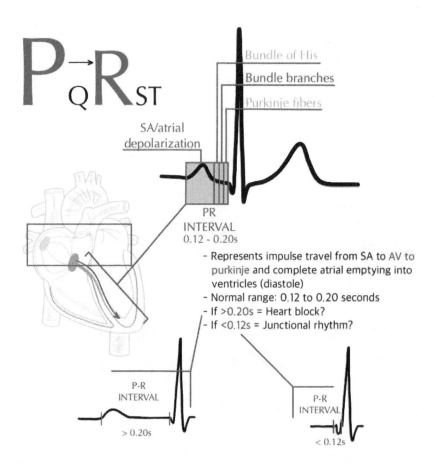

Following (and encompassing) the P wave, is the PR interval.

What is the PR interval?

This part of the cardiac cycle includes the time needed for atrial depolarization and ends with depolarization through the AV node and all the way to the purkinje system[19]. It should be *constant* in length and between 0.12 and 0.20 seconds[21].

What does this mean?

During this time, the atria are fully contracting and emptying into the ventricles. The iso-electric (flat) P-R (sometimes PQ) *Segment* following the P wave allows for *complete atrial emptying and ventricular filling* before progression to the QRS complex (ventricular activation). What's essentially happening is the impulse is rapidly travelling all the way through to the purkinje fibers even though these events aren't large enough to produce visible changes on the surface ECG. Once this impulse activates and spreads through enough of the ventricular myocardium, our QRS then becomes evident, representing ventricular depolarization[19].

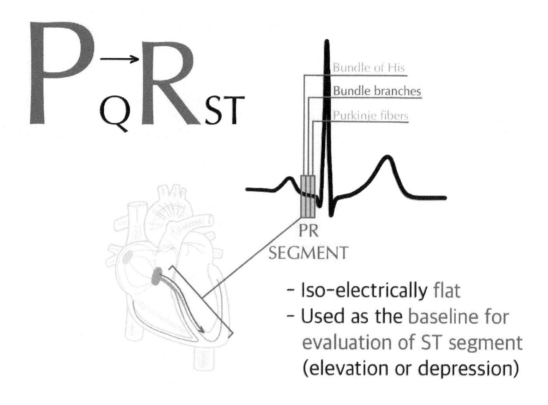

PR SEGMENT

- Iso-electrically flat
- Used as the baseline for evaluation of ST segment (elevation or depression)

The P-R *interval* should be between 0.12 and 0.20 seconds. If it's less than 0.12 seconds the impulse may be junctional, may represent a low atrial origin, or sinus origin with ventricular pre-excitation, among other conditions. The P wave may be upright, inverted, or non-existent. But how could the P wave possibly be non-existent? If the P wave is inverted, it may be before the QRS or right after the QRS. If it's nowhere to be found it's likely to be *hidden* within the QRS, but it's still there.

Let's think back to *Rule #1 of interpreting basic cardiac rhythms*: understanding that an impulse traveling *toward a positive* electrode will produce a *positive (upward) deflection.* If your impulse is starting downstream (like in the vicinity of the AV junction) then it will have to travel *backward*, upstream to activate the part of the upper atria for which the SA node was originally responsible. This is called *retrograde* (backward) conduction.

And if Rule #1 is that a *positive* impulse travelling toward a *positive* electrode produces a *positive* (upright) deflection, then a positive impulse travelling *away* from a positive electrode should produce a *negative* deflection. Therefore *inverted* P waves are said to be junctional if the PR interval is short (<0.12s)[17]; they originate from the AV junction and travel backward while the rest of the impulse heads toward the ventricles as it usually would. Think of it as sending a messenger to the upper atria while you continue to head toward the ventricles using the normal conduction fast track. Inverted P waves with a normal PR interval are suggestive of ectopic atrial origin. Junctional P waves are covered in greater detail in Chapter 7.

If the P-R interval is greater than 0.20 seconds, you may be looking at an atrio-ventricular block (AVB), meaning that for some reason the impulse is taking its sweet time to reach the ventricles. The P-R interval may be long and constant with 1:1 atrial to ventricular conduction (1st degree AV block), variable and lengthening with ensuing beats (2nd degree type 1 AV block), or in total disconnect and unrelated to the QRS (complete/3rd degree AVB). We'll cover these in depth in Chapter 9.

Why should we care?

The P-R interval provides clues as to where atrial and junctional beats are originating and what the relationship is between those beats and the ventricles below. This can all be inferred based upon the time relationship between the two. Next up let's look at the QRS complex and ventricular activation.

TAKE HOME POINTS

✓ The PR interval describes the time needed for the impulse to leave the SA node, arrive at the AV node, and complete propagation through to the purkinje network
✓ The PR interval should be *constant* in length and between 0.12 and 0.20 seconds.
✓ Less than 0.12 seconds *may* indicate a junctional rhythm
✓ Greater than 0.20 seconds may indicate an AV block or impulse delay
✓ Inverted P waves indicate retrograde (backward) atrial conduction

The QRS complex

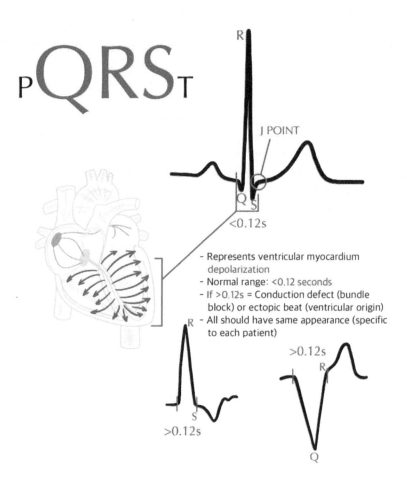

What is the QRS complex?

The QRS complex represents ventricular depolarization.

What does this mean?

This complex is short in duration (< 0.12 seconds)[13] largely thanks to the purkinje fibers, where the impulse picks up a lot of speed. This is important since the ventricles are relatively thick and need to depolarize simultaneously to allow as much blood as possible to be expelled.

In cases where the QRS complex is greater than 0.12 seconds, the ventricles are taking longer to depolarize which is inefficient. If it's a single, early, wide beat on the ECG, it may be a premature ventricular contraction (PVC). If they come as 3 or more successively, you may be looking at ventricular tachycardia, a potentially lethal rhythm if sustained (aberrant bundle branch block conduction may also cause this but is beyond this scope). With sustained inefficient beats at a high rate, ejection fraction may decrease, ventricular filling time may reduce, cardiac output might decrease, and blood supply to the heart via the coronary arteries may also decreasing during diastole.

Why should I care?

Rapid rates with a wide cardiac conduction time also may increase the oxygen demand on the heart leading to ischemia, potential myocardial injury, and patient deterioration. Understanding why a narrow QRS is important as well as the ability to recognize a wide QRS will help in appreciating the importance of frequent wide and bizarre looking complexes when analyzing rhythm strips in the future.

TAKE HOME POINTS

- ✓ The QRS complex represents ventricular depolarization
- ✓ The QRS should measure < 0.12 seconds
- ✓ Wide QRS complexes may represent inefficiency
- ✓ Wide ventricular origin rhythms at a very rapid rate may be lethal if sustained and negatively affecting hemodynamic stability

The J point and ST segment

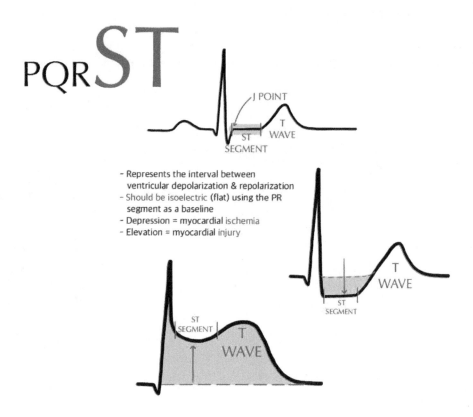

- Represents the interval between ventricular depolarization & repolarization
- Should be isoelectric (flat) using the PR segment as a baseline
- Depression = myocardial ischemia
- Elevation = myocardial injury

What is the ST segment?

Following the QRS complex is the ST segment. Before looking at this diagnostic segment we should first understand the *J point*. The J point is the point at which the S wave of the QRS makes the turn to head back to baseline (J joins the S with the T). This is important because this marks the beginning of the ST segment.

The normal ST segment should be flat (isoelectric) at baseline. This can be evaluated by using the PR segment (or sometimes the P-Q junction with rapid heart rates) as the isoelectric starting point. To evaluate if the ST segment falls above, in line, or below the PR segment draw a straight, horizontal line from one to the other (note some sources may cite the TP segment as baseline although this may not be possible at higher rates, as time between cardiac cycles is decreased. From a nursing standpoint, the PR segment or PQ junction would be acceptable)[17,22].

What does this mean?

From a strictly ischemic standpoint, ST segment depression may represent myocardial ischemia (impaired oxygen delivery). ST segment elevation may warn of potential tissue injury and tissue death if untreated (the *STEMI*; ST elevation myocardial infarction). Broadly speaking, the injury is likely to hurt you first (elevation), but both should be treated with respect since each may rapidly progress to deterioration. Of course, many conditions may cause ST segment depression (such as left ventricular strain pattern) and elevation (benign early repolarization, Brugada syndrome, etc.). Regardless, grab a prior ECG for comparison if available and treat the patient, not solely the monitor. The monitor is there to provide context to the overall clinical picture.

ST segment elevation and depression are described partly in terms of millimeters. At paper speed of 25 mm/sec, the smallest box on the ECG paper is 0.04 seconds in duration, and 1mm in length and height.

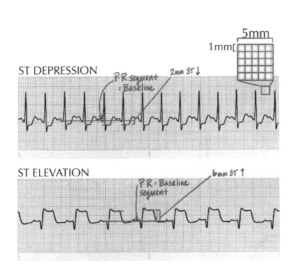 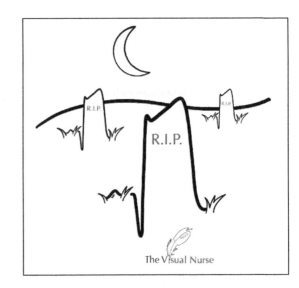

Tombstoning ST elevation (bottom left; right) describes a distinct form of ST elevation that's associated with poor prognosis if not corrected quickly[23].

Why should we care?

The ST segment is one of the strongest diagnostic considerations when a patient is experiencing chest pain or other veiled symptoms. Women and diabetics in particular may not always report chest pain as anginal equivalents, however. Nausea, jaw pain, dyspnea, fatigue, and other symptoms may be ominous presentations that should be clinically correlated with ECG findings[10]. Symptomatic ST changes must be treated accordingly, and the pain must resolve completely. The key is to compare to a previous ECG when possible and to collect serial ECGs which may show trends over time.

TAKE HOME POINTS

- ✓ The J point is the point at which the S wave of the QRS makes the turn to head back to baseline and marks the beginning of the ST segment
- ✓ The normal ST segment should be flat (isoelectric) and in line with the PR segment
- ✓ ST segment depression may indicate myocardial ischemia
- ✓ ST segment elevation may indicate myocardial injury

The T wave

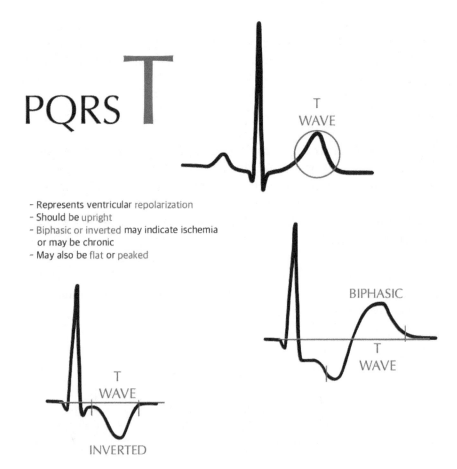

PQRS **T**

T WAVE

- Represents ventricular repolarization
- Should be upright
- Biphasic or inverted may indicate ischemia
  or may be chronic
- May also be flat or peaked

BIPHASIC

T WAVE

T WAVE

INVERTED

What is the T wave?

The T wave represents ventricular repolarization and is a relatively slower process than that of ventricular depolarization[19]. This manifests as a broader and smoother waveform as compared to the QRS.

What does this mean?

At this point the ventricles are repolarizing, meaning they're unable to respond to incoming impulses. The cells of the heart are in the process of recharging for the next impulse and wave of contraction. Sometimes, you may see a premature atrial complex (P wave) delivered and the ventricles will not respond. It can sometimes mimic a transient heart block so take a closer look at the P – P interval. Essentially the ventricles are saying, "Sorry, we're on break, so send another sinus beat in a few seconds and we'll pick that one up."

I like to compare this repolarization state to the windshield wipers on your car. When the wipers are in the down-swing process of wiping, if you decide to bump the wiper signal to clear the windshield one more time, do the wipers stop halfway and automatically go back up? Not typically. They travel all the way back to resting before completing the next sweep that you signaled. This illustrates the concept of refractoriness and is one significance of the T wave: signifying the repolarization of the ventricles to their resting state in preparation for the next signal.

We have not discussed the QT interval yet but as a preface to the next section, in cases where the QT interval is prolonged, an early PVC or other beat has the potential to land on the T wave during a vulnerable period. If this happens the heart can be sent into a beautiful but potentially lethal rhythm known as *Torsades de pointes* (Chapter 8).

Why should we care?

T waves should be upright (exceptions exist on the 12-lead ECG). Abnormal T waves may be peaked, flat, inverted, or biphasic (meaning they're below and above the isoelectric line). Tall, peaked T waves may represent electrolyte abnormalities, most commonly hyperkalemia (hyper = high, kalemia = potassium in the blood). Flat, inverted, or biphasic T waves may represent myocardial ischemia. They may also be chronic in some conditions and conduction abnormalities. In any case, assess the patient and obtain a prior ECG for comparison if possible.

The first ECG below shows a sinus bradycardia with biphasic T waves. The second ECG depicts inverted T waves in a rhythm showing sinus bradycardia with a first-degree AV delay. Remember, if this is a change from baseline, T wave inversion may represent possible ischemia until confirmed otherwise[13].

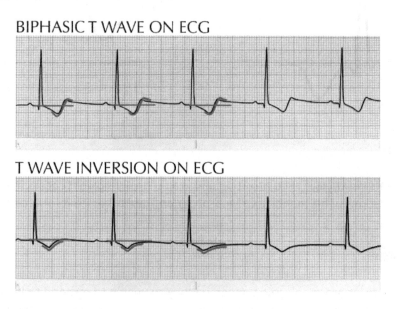

BIPHASIC T WAVE ON ECG

T WAVE INVERSION ON ECG

TAKE HOME POINTS:

- ✓ The T wave represents ventricular repolarization
- ✓ Abnormal T waves may be peaked, flat, inverted, or biphasic
- ✓ Flat or inverted T waves may represent myocardial ischemia; assess the patient and correlate with the clinical picture

The QT interval

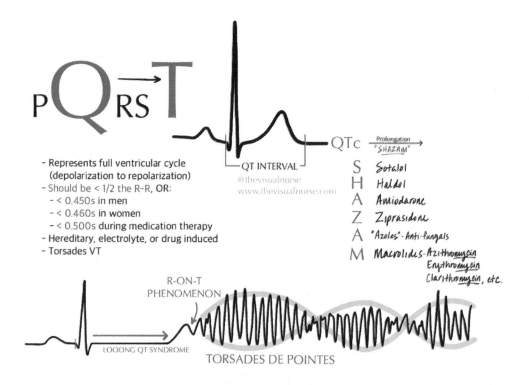

- Represents full ventricular cycle
  (depolarization to repolarization)
- Should be < 1/2 the R-R, OR:
  - < 0.450s in men
  - < 0.460s in women
  - < 0.500s during medication therapy
- Hereditary, electrolyte, or drug induced
- Torsades VT

QT INTERVAL
@thevisualnurse
www.thevisualnurse.com

QTc — Prolongation → "SHAZAM"
S Sotalol
H Haldol
A Amiodarone
Z Ziprasidone
A "Azoles"- Anti-fungals
M Macrolides-Azithromycin
   Erythromycin
   Clarithromycin, etc.

R-ON-T PHENOMENON

LOOONG QT SYNDROME

TORSADES DE POINTES

What is the QT interval?

The QT interval (QTI) represents a single *ventricular* cycle of depolarization and repolarization.

What does this mean?

If you recall the previous letters of the cardiac cycle and what each represent, this will tell you exactly what the QT interval is describing. The "Q" of the QRS complex represents the beginning of ventricular myocardium depolarization. The T wave represents ventricular repolarization. Together, the QTI describes the time the entire process takes.

Speaking of time, what are the acceptable intervals for this measure? Broadly, the QT interval should be less than half the R-to-R interval. More specifically, the QTI should be ≤ 0.45 seconds in men, and ≤ 0.46 seconds in women. Each 0.010s (10 millisecond) increase in QT interval corrected for heart rate (QTc) was found to be associated with an increase in instance of heart failure, cardiovascular events, and stroke of 25%, 11% and 19%, respectively, at an 8 year follow up period[13].

Why should we care?

Long QT syndrome may be hereditary, electrolyte induced, or drug induced. Medications with antiarrhythmic properties like Sotalol, Flecainide, Amiodarone, and others have the potential to prolong this interval. Patients undergoing loading therapies for these drug types are often have their QT intervals monitored using serial ECGs. If you notice a QT interval approaching or exceeding 0.500 seconds in these patients, notify the provider *as per physician orders and established workplace guidelines*. The provider should specify measurement guidelines for which they'd like to be notified.

Left untreated, long QT syndrome predisposes patient to a potentially lethal form of ventricular tachycardia known as *Torsades de Pointes* ("twisting of the points"; Chapter 8) which may occur if a PVC or other early beat strikes the T wave while the ventricles are refractory (there's that word again..) If this happens, the heart is thrown into an electrically chaotic state where cardiac output may fall dramatically if sustained. Remember, cardiac arrhythmias are largely about the effect they have on cardiac output. On the next page you'll find a (not-conclusive) list of medications known to commonly prolong the QT interval. Be on the lookout for these!

TAKE HOME (Torsades de) **POINTES:**

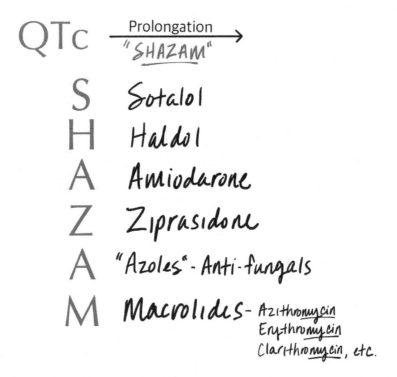

QTc Prolongation →
"SHAZAM"

S Sotalol
H Haldol
A Amiodarone
Z Ziprasidone
A "Azoles"- Anti-fungals
M Macrolides- Azithromycin
       Erythromycin
       Clarithromycin, etc.

✓ The QT interval (QTI) represents a single *ventricular* cycle of depolarization and repolarization
✓ The QT interval should be either 1) less than half the R - R interval 2) ≤ 0.45 seconds in men or 3) ≤ 0.46 seconds in women
✓ Long QT syndrome may predispose patients to a potentially lethal form of ventricular tachycardia known as *Torsades de Pointes*
✓ Long QT syndrome may be hereditary, electrolyte induced, or drug induced

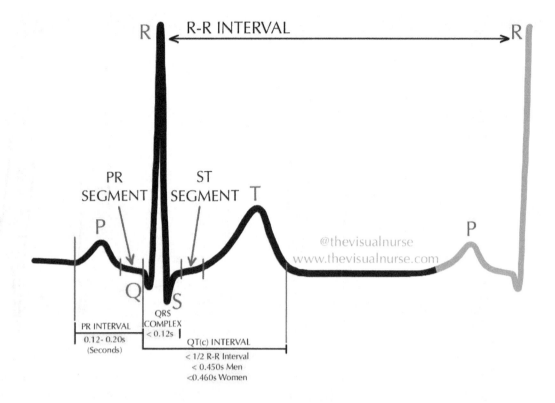

This is the same image we saw at the beginning of the chapter. I hope we were able to tie each concept together sufficiently enough that you now see the story that the cardiac cycle tells. You should bookmark this page for later use as a quick reference.

TAKE HOME POINTS:

✓ Easily remember the norms for cardiac cycle intervals: 12 to 20 (PRI), less than 12 (QRS), add all three to get 44 or less (QT).

CHAPTER 4: HOW DO WE STANDARDIZE RHYTHMS?

USING CALIPERS

To measure waveforms

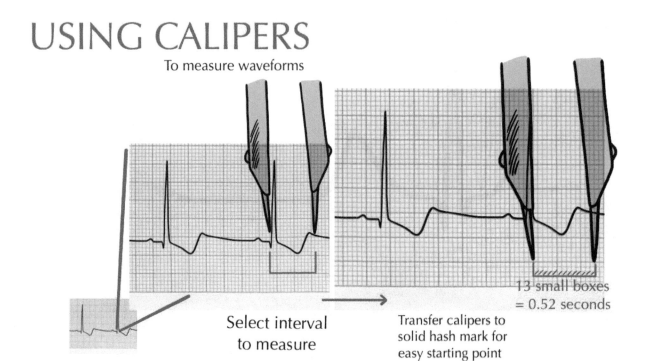

Select interval
to measure

Transfer calipers to
solid hash mark for
easy starting point

13 small boxes
= 0.52 seconds

Special paper for waveform recording

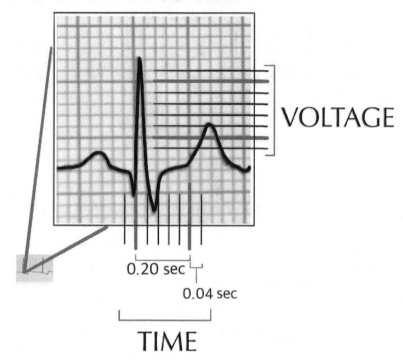

What is ECG paper?

Electrocardiography graph paper is a standardized tool. It uses time as a constant variable so that rhythms can be identified accurately and compared against one another. Voltage is a constant as well, but the focus here is on the grid as it relates to time. If you progress from basic rhythm interpretation to 12-lead ECG interpretation, voltage will be discussed in greater detail.

What does this mean?

Why are some lines thick and some narrow? What do they mean? Before we can describe anything regarding the naming or classification of a rhythm, we must know that the intervals have been compared against a standardized backdrop. This is what the ECG paper provides.

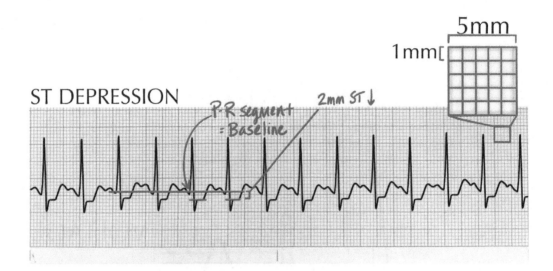

The "smallest box" on the paper with the *thin* pink (or sometimes grey) lines measures 0.04 seconds (4 one-hundredths of a second). The "big box" with the *thick*er line measures 0.20 seconds (2 tenths of a second). If you're a math whiz, you'll notice there are 5 small boxes in one big box. You'll also notice that 30 of these big boxes are equal to 6 seconds (0.20 X 30 = 6 seconds). Trust me, I hate math too. The reason I mention this is, typically when you're being tested on simple rhythm analysis, you'll be shown a 6 second strip that's running at 25 millimeters per second (mm/s)[22].

Now, you've also probably figured out that if you count the total QRS complexes in a 6 second strip and multiply by 10 (6 seconds X 10 = 60 seconds = 1 minute) you'll know the heart rate in terms of *beats per minute*. And I've yet to see heart rate presented in any format other than *beats per minute*.

Why should we care?

Sure, you can look at a rhythm strip and notice that there is one P wave per QRS complex and that the R waves seems to be marching out on time, but what if I showed you a rhythm strip with no ECG graph lines? Would you be able to identify a first-degree AV block? Would you be able to say beyond a shadow of a doubt that you were looking at a normal sinus rhythm and not sinus or other atrial tachycardia? Of course, you could guess, but to make the proper call you need an absolute constant that is true from rhythm to rhythm. Time is that constant and it's why we use standardized paper with known variables. Now, what's the easiest way to count and measure all these boxes? Check out the next section on measuring wave forms to find out.

TAKE HOME POINTS

- ✓ ECG graph paper is a standardized tool that uses time as a constant variable
- ✓ The smallest box measures 0.04 seconds and the "big box" measures 0.20 seconds
- ✓ There are 5 small boxes in each big box
- ✓ 30 "big" (0.20 second) boxes equal 6 seconds which is how most rhythm strips are presented for testing purposes

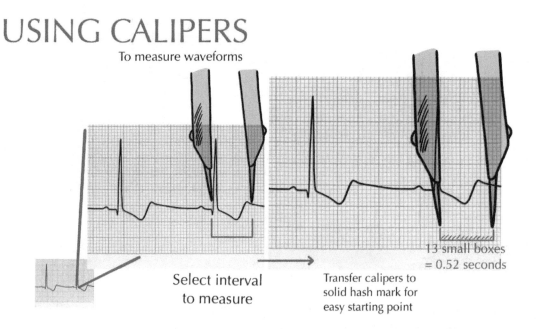

USING CALIPERS
To measure waveforms

Select interval
to measure

Transfer calipers to
solid hash mark for
easy starting point

13 small boxes
= 0.52 seconds

What are calipers?

Calipers are handheld tools that allow simple and rapid measurement of ECG intervals. Standardized measurements are necessary for naming and classifying cardiac rhythms.

What does this mean?

To measure the interval(s) of interest quickly and accurately, we follow two easy steps. Step 1: select the interval to be measured and place your caliper points on the nearest line. Step 2: transfer your calipers somewhere on the ECG paper so that the first point lands on the hash mark of a "big (0.20 second) box." This provides an easy starting point to follow when we count the number of boxes between caliper points.

Why should we care?

Often, you'll be able to simply look at the PR interval and notice that it extends beyond 0.20 seconds. Other times however, it may be difficult to differentiate your intervals without assistance. For example, with rapid atrial fibrillation rates approaching 180 to 200 beats per minute, it can be very difficult to tell if the R waves are regular or irregularly spaced. In many cases, a pair of calipers will help with differentiation.

Do your P waves appear to be in discord with your QRS complexes? Grab your calipers and you may notice that you're looking at a complete heart block if differing atrial and ventricular rates are present with a PR interval that varies for each beat. Making the right call on a rhythm makes a big difference in patient care. If you don't have a set of calipers handy, you can always use the paper method in a pinch.

PAPER METHOD
Of measuring waveforms

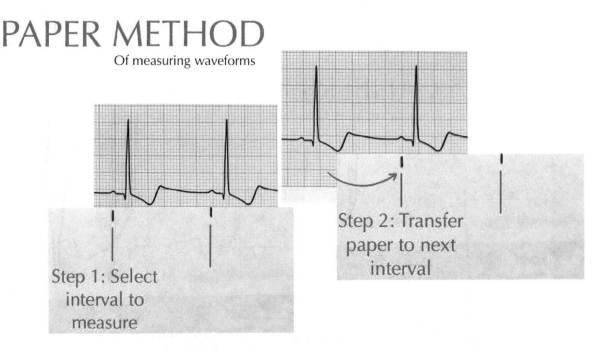

Step 1: Select interval to measure

Step 2: Transfer paper to next interval

The paper method can also be used to determine if a rhythm is regular or irregular (if the P waves and R waves march out routinely) if you don't have a set of calipers nearby. Simply make hash marks on your paper corresponding with the waveform of interest, then slide the paper to the next waveform in line to determine if the complexes land on the same hash marks. Like the caliper method on the previous page, this method can also be used to obtain *measurements* of specific intervals if needed. Now that we've introduced the tools we use for rhythm determination, we need a consistent method for approaching each rhythm strip.

TAKE HOME POINTS

- ✓ Calipers allow for rapid interval determination
- ✓ First, select the interval to be measured and place your caliper points on the nearest corresponding lines
- ✓ Next, transfer your calipers so that the first point lands on the hash mark of a "big (0.20 second) box" and count the total boxes between the points
- ✓ The paper method can also be used to determine waveform regularity or interval measurements if you don't have a pair of calipers present

Standardizing rhythm evaluation

1. RATE: Atrial: _____   Ventricular: _____
2. RHYTHM: <u>Atrial</u> Regular Irregular   <u>Ventricular</u> Regular Irregular
3. P WAVES: _____ 4. PR: _____ 5. QRS: _____ 6. QT:
7. ST SEGMENT: Okay Elevated Depressed   8. T WAVES: _____

What is rhythm analysis?

This is the 8-step rhythm analysis format that I use every day. The absolute key to learning rhythm analysis is using the same stepwise progression every single time. This prevents us from becoming overwhelmed when we encounter a rhythm strip that resembles a Richter scale printout. Of course, with practice, your eyes will learn to quickly skim and summarize these steps as second nature but first, we should build the foundation that allows us to train our eyes over time.

Rhythm analysis can resemble a tangled mess of wires (like the ones you pull out of your attic each year around the holidays) or it can take on the appearance of the clean, streamlined, and labelled wires associated with a well organized commercial computer server system. It's up to you.

What does this mean?

Ultimately, *you* will decide how difficult or easy rhythm interpretation will be. It's up to you to practice and use this process daily until you can repeat it without thinking. I recommend doing at least one sample rhythm strip each day using this approach. Set a daily timer if you need to. It should only take 5 minutes of your day but by doing so, your axe will become a little sharper with each strip that you see and eventually your eyes will begin to read the strips as you're reading this paragraph. Remember, long term consistency beats short term intensity and practice makes perfect.

Why should we care?

How do we keep from getting tangled up? Say the following with me: **"R, P, and Q times two (x2)... STAT!"** This mnemonic describes the progression that we'll follow. If you're visual like me, here's an illustrative example...

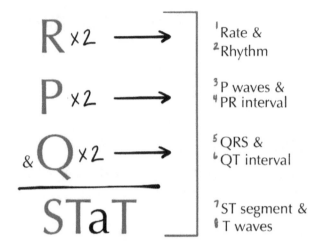

"R, P, and Q times two (x2)... STAT!"

Rate: What's the heart rate in beats per minute?

Rhythm (regularity): Is the rhythm regular or irregular, meaning "Do the P waves and QRS complexes march out routinely?"

P waves: Are they present? What's the appearance?

PR: What does the PR interval measure?

QRS: What does the QRS interval measure? Is it narrow or wide?

QT: What does the QT interval measure?

ST: Is the ST segment elevated, depressed, or in line with the PR segment?

T: Are they normal and upright or are they abnormal (peaked, flat, inverted, or biphasic)?

The trick is to follow the same process each time when first learning rhythm interpretation. Don't be lured into getting tangled up in all the information that a rhythm strip provides by jumping to step 6. Don't step over nickels to pick up pennies. Sharpen your axe daily.

TAKE HOME POINTS:

- ✓ The key to learning rhythm analysis is using the same progression every time
- ✓ Practice at least one sample rhythm strip each day using the same approach
- ✓ Remember RPQ x 2 STaT: Rate & Rhythm, P & PR, QRS & QT, ST & T
- ✓ Read on to find out how each is determined

Step 1: Calculating heart rate

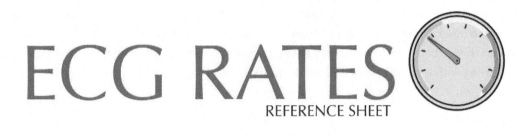

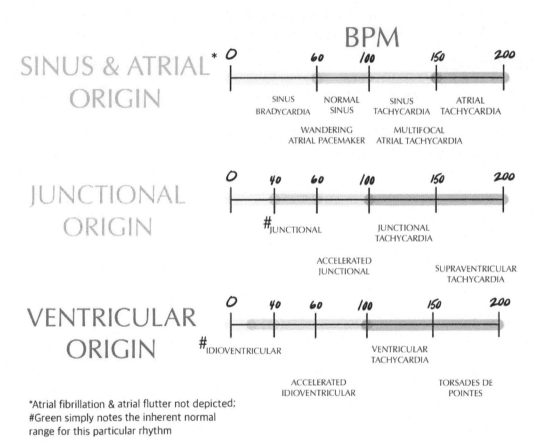

*Atrial fibrillation & atrial flutter not depicted;
#Green simply notes the inherent normal
range for this particular rhythm

**Supraventricular tachycardia in this image and subsequent copies refers to paroxysmal SVT (PSVT), commonly atrioventricular nodal re-entrant tachycardias (AVNRT) and atrio-ventricular tachycardias (AVRT). Rates may range 100 – 250+ but are commonly >150 beats per minute.*

What is heart rate?

Heart rate describes how fast the heart is beating. It's standardized in terms of beats per minute. The image above provides an overview of heart rates as they relate to each site of rhythm origin. As we progress, we'll cover each location in detail.

What does this mean?

Together with clinical presentation, heart rates guide the assessment and treatment of patients. One of the most important concepts related to heart rate is the effect it has on cardiac output (CO = HR X SV). As heart rate increases so does cardiac output...to a certain point. The heart feeds itself with oxygen-rich blood using the coronary arteries during *diastole*. At a certain point if heart rate is too fast, the heart has less and less time to spend in diastole which means the ability of the coronary arteries to feed the heart decreases. When this is the case, demand may exceed supply. There's a big difference in cardiac output when you're dealing with a heart rate of 150 BPM versus 350 BPM when ventricular filling is compromised.

Why should we care?

Our ability to rapidly determine heart rate will result in quicker responses and interventions that are appropriate. Read on to discover three common methods for determining heart rate.

TAKE HOME POINTS:

- ✓ Heart rate describes how fast the heart is beating and is standardized in terms of beats per minute
- ✓ Cardiac output increases as heart rate increases to a finite degree
- ✓ Extremely rapid heart rates may impair diastolic filling time resulting in decreased cardiac output

Step 1:

RATE: The 6 second method

RATE: Atrial: _____   Ventricular: _____
RHYTHM: <u>Atrial</u> Regular Irregular   <u>Ventricular</u> Regular Irregular
P WAVES: _____   PR: _____   QRS: _____   QT: _____
ST SEGMENT: Okay Elevated Depressed   T WAVES: _____

What is the 6 second method?

The 6 second method is a common and simple way to evaluate heart rate. This is the preferred method when first learning rhythm interpretation since most exams will present sample strips in this way. Of course, all three methods that we're going to look at in this section have their own advantages and disadvantages.

What does this mean?

The 6 second method refers to the timing of our rhythm strip. Find the red hash marks in the example above. Remember from our conversation earlier on ECG graph paper that 30 big (0.20 second) boxes equal 6 seconds. Once you've confirmed you have a 6 second rhythm strip the rest is easy!

What's the heart rate for the rhythm above? If you said 110 beats per minute, well done (11 QRS complexes x 10 = 110 BPM)!

Why should we care?

For testing purposes, most rhythm strips will be presented as a 6 second strip. This method is one of the simplest and quickest for determining heart rate. In a 6 second strip like the one shown (note the bottom pink markers), count the total QRS complexes (ventricular beats). Next, multiply by 10 (6 seconds x 10 = 60 seconds = 1 minute). That's it! Do the same for the P waves. Remember, *there should only be one P wave for each QRS complex.* Let's look at two more methods of determining heart rate next.

TAKE HOME POINTS:

- ✓ The 6 second method for determining heart rate is the preferred method when first learning rhythm interpretation since most exams will present sample strips in this way
- ✓ For a 6 second strip count the total QRS complexes and multiply by 10 to arrive at the heart rate. That's it! Do the same for the P waves

Heart rate: the small box method

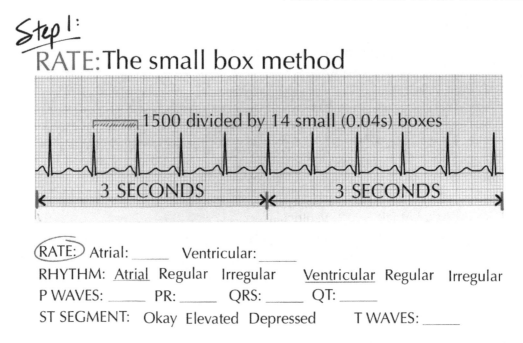

Step 1:

RATE: The small box method

1500 divided by 14 small (0.04s) boxes

3 SECONDS   3 SECONDS

RATE: Atrial: _____   Ventricular: _____
RHYTHM: Atrial Regular Irregular   Ventricular Regular Irregular
P WAVES: _____   PR: _____   QRS: _____   QT: _____
ST SEGMENT: Okay Elevated Depressed   T WAVES: _____

What is the small box method?

The small box method is another common and simple way to evaluate heart rate.

What does this mean?

To use the small box method for calculating heart rate find an R wave, ideally one that resides on a solid line. Mark the very next R wave that you see. Now, count the number of small boxes (clever!) between each R wave. Divide 1500 by the number of small boxes between R waves to arrive at the heart rate! The rate for the strip above would be 107 BPM (1500 / 14 = 107).

Why does this method work? I'm glad you asked. Remember that ECG paper is a standardized backdrop that uses time as a constant. Let's review a few concepts:

- ✓ Each smallest box on our ECG paper measures 0.04 seconds (at 25mm/s)
- ✓ We're interested in heart rate as a function of beats *per minute*
- ✓ There are 60 seconds in each minute
- ✓ This means there are 1500 small boxes in *each minute* (because 60 seconds divided by 0.04 equals 1500)
- ✓ So if we divide 1500 (representing 1 minute) by the amount of small boxes between each beat, we can figure out how many of these beats are occurring *each minute*. Pretty cool!

Why should we care?

The advantage to the small box method is that it gives a much more precise rate count than the 6 second method although it takes slightly more time. The major disadvantage to the small box method is that it should only be used for *regular rhythms* (more on this later) since the number of small boxes is constant between R waves. Comparatively, the number of small boxes will fluctuate between beats in an irregular rhythm. Of course, you could find the range of small boxes between each of the R waves in an irregular rhythm but who wants to torture themselves with that?

TAKE HOME POINTS:

- ✓ The small box method provides a more accurate heart rate measure for regular rhythms than the 6 second method
- ✓ To do this, count the number of small boxes between each R wave and divide 1500 by the number of small boxes to arrive at the heart rate

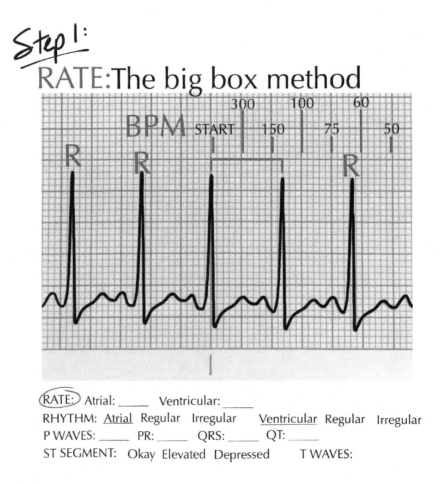

Step 1:
RATE: The big box method

CRATE: Atrial: _____ Ventricular: _____
RHYTHM: <u>Atrial</u> Regular Irregular   <u>Ventricular</u> Regular Irregular
P WAVES: _____ PR: _____ QRS: _____ QT: _____
ST SEGMENT: Okay Elevated Depressed   T WAVES:

What is the big box method?

The big box method is the third common way to evaluate heart rate.

What does this mean?

Using the big box method for calculating heart rate involves some degree of memorization.

✓ Before you begin, memorize the following 6 numbers: "300, 150, 100... 75, 60, 50."

Next, find an R wave that resides on a *thick (0.20 second) solid* line. With each "big box" line that comes, count off the numbers, "300, 150, 100... 75, 60, 50." In the example above, the second R wave from the "start"-ing line falls between 100 and 150 beats per minute. You've probably already guessed that the disadvantage to this method is its lack of precision relative to the small box method. The overwhelming advantage is the rapid determination of heart rate the big box method allows.

As with the small box method, the big box method works using time as a constant variable:

- ✓ Each big box on our ECG paper measures 0.20 seconds
- ✓ We're interested in heart rate as a function of beats *per minute*
- ✓ There are 60 seconds in each minute
- ✓ This means there are 300 big boxes in *each minute* (because 60 seconds divided by 0.20 equals 300 beats *per minute* if an R wave were to fall exactly on each big box line)
- ✓ If an R wave were to fall on every *other* big box line, this equals a beat occurring every 0.40 seconds (0.20 x 2). Now, 60 seconds divided by 0.40 equals 150 beats *per minute* if an R wave were to fall exactly every *other* big box line. See the pattern?

Why should we care?

Again, the resounding advantage to the big box method is that it allows for very rapid approximation of heart rates. This is important when decisions need to be made quickly and a heart rate approximation is all that's needed. Clearly the advantage the first two methods have over this method is a more acute rate determination for the reasons mentioned above. This wraps up rate determination. Next up is regularity!

TAKE HOME POINTS:

- ✓ The big box method allows for rapid approximation of heart rate when quick decisions are needed
- ✓ Commit the following numbers to memory: 300, 150, 100 ... 75, 60, 50

Step 2: Rhythm regularity

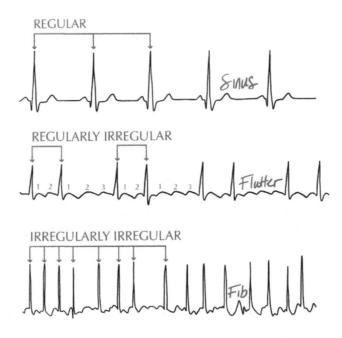

What is rhythm regularity?

Regularity indicates the presence of an identifiable pattern. Rhythm regularity is the term used to describe this. What is the pattern of the electrical activity? Is there no pattern at all? Do the atrial and ventricular beats come on time as expected with each beat or are there unexpected distances (time) between them?

What does this mean?

Remember there should be one P wave per QRS (atrial depolarization per ventricular depolarization). The simplest way to determine regularity is to ask yourself, "Are the waves the same distance apart?" If the answer is yes, it's *regular*. If not, it's *irregular*. That's it! Be sure to do this from P wave to P wave *and* R wave to R wave.

Why should we care?

The ability to identify regularity or irregularity will allow you to quickly *exclude* particular rhythms in order to arrive at the correct interpretation much faster.

Step 2

RHYTHM (Regularity): Are P-P & R-R same distance apart?

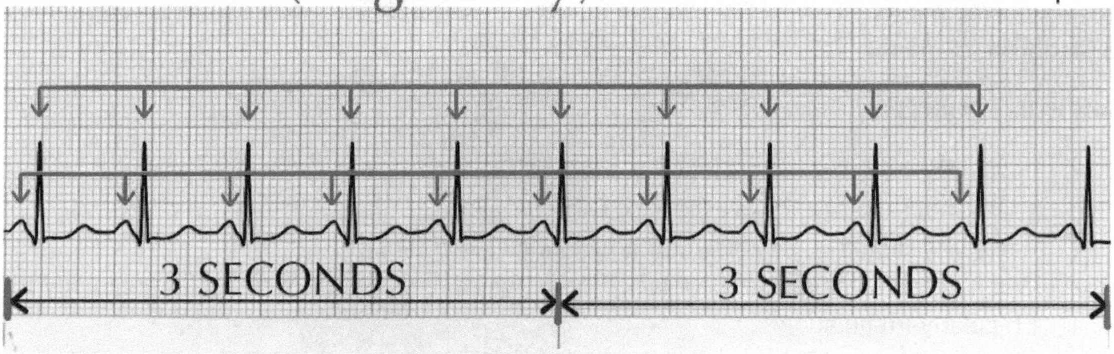

RATE: Atrial: _100_   Ventricular: _100_

(RHYTHM) Atrial (Regular) Irregular   Ventricular (Regular) Irregular

P WAVES: _____   PR: _____   QRS: _____   QT: _____

ST SEGMENT: Okay Elevated Depressed   T WAVES: _____

When determining regularity or lack thereof we have three options:

- ✓ Regular
- ✓ Regularly irregular
- ✓ Irregularly irregular

Step 2

REGULARITY

REGULAR

(i.e. Normal Sinus Rhythm)

IRREGULAR

REGULARLY IRREGULAR

(i.e. Some forms of Atrial Flutter)

IRREGULARLY IRREGULAR

(i.e. Atrial Fibrillation)

Regularity should be described individually for both atrial and ventricular activity. Regular rhythms indicate that our P's and QRS are coming on time each time as expected.

Irregular rhythms may or may not have an identifiable pattern. If our QRS vary in the distance (time) between beats but seem to do so in a rhythmic pattern, we classify them as *regularly* irregular. If our QRS vary in the distance (time) between beats and offer no identifiable pattern, we classify them as *irregularly* irregular. We'll dive a little deeper into this during our discussion on atrial flutter and atrial fibrillation in Chapter 6.

TAKE HOME POINTS:

- ✓ Regularity indicates the presence of an identifiable pattern
- ✓ There should be one P wave for each QRS complex
- ✓ Regularity should be described for both P waves and QRS
- ✓ When determining regularity or lack thereof we have three options: Regular, regularly-irregular, irregularly-irregular

Putting the puzzle together

SAMPLE INTERPRETATION

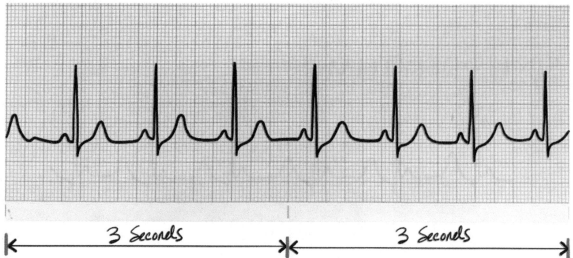

RATE: Atrial: _70_ Ventricular: _70_ (6 second method)

RHYTHM: Atrial (Regular) Irregular   Ventricular (Regular) Irregular

P WAVES: _Upright_ PR: _0.16_ QRS: _0.06_ QT: _0.40_

ST SEGMENT: (Okay) Elevated Depressed   T WAVES: _Upright_

FINAL INTERPRETATION: _Normal sinus rhythm_

How do we put it all together?

Everything we've covered together to point has led us to the final interpretation of our rhythm strip. Following steps number 1 and 2, complete your measurements and interpretations for all segments of the cardiac cycle that we learned previously and watch the puzzle begin to come together.

What does this mean?

Use the formatted template above to jot down your rate, rhythm regularity, segments, and intervals.

Why should we care?

This template will help train your mind to work through each rhythm methodically. With enough repetition you'll be able to lose the training wheels and work through this progression naturally.

TAKE HOME POINTS:

✓ That's it! Now you have the tools to begin breaking down your rhythm strips. So, let's get to them!

CHAPTER 5: RHYTHMS AND ARRHYTHMIAS OF SINUS ORIGIN

SINUS RHYTHM

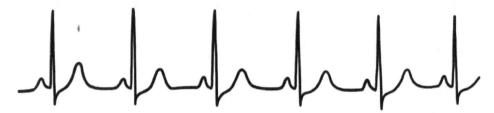

SINUS BRADYCARDIA

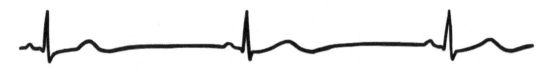

SINUS TACHYCARDIA

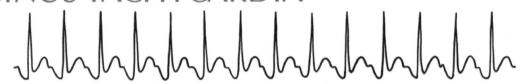

SINUS ARRHYTHMIA

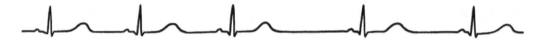

SINUS ORIGIN

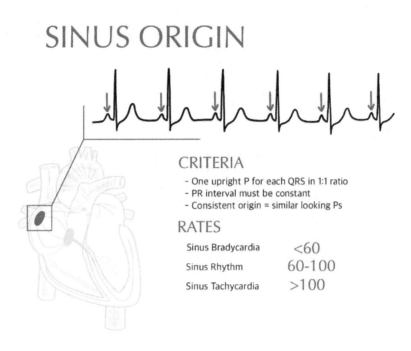

CRITERIA
- One upright P for each QRS in 1:1 ratio
- PR interval must be constant
- Consistent origin = similar looking Ps

RATES

Sinus Bradycardia	<60
Sinus Rhythm	60-100
Sinus Tachycardia	>100

What is sinus origin?

A rhythm of sinus origin describes an impulse that originates at the SA node.

What does this mean?

This group of rhythms maintains specific criteria. There should be one upright P wave for each QRS, the PR interval should be constant, and all P waves should be similar in appearance. Sinus rhythm describes the normal conduction pathway, beginning with the SA node and terminating in the ventricles in a 1:1 fashion.

If the PR interval is inconsistent, it's possible there may be a conduction abnormality present known as an *atrioventricular block*. The fact that the PR interval is constant means the impulse is taking the same time to travel from the SA node to the ventricles with each beat.

Why should we care?

All P waves should look the same. Remember that all cardiac cells possess a degree of automaticity (under particular circumstances) meaning that they may spontaneously discharge. If all P waves look the same, *we assume them to be sinus*, coming from the sino-atrial node[13]. If P waves differ in appearance this tells us that there are impulses originating somewhere else the atria in addition to our normal P waves, but they probably *aren't sinus*. We've touched on this concept earlier in the case of the wandering atrial pacemaker which we'll revisit in Chapter 6.

TAKE HOME POINTS:

- ✓ The sinus origin rhythms describe an impulse that originates at the SA node
- ✓ There should only be one upright P wave for each QRS in a 1:1 ratio with similar appearing P waves
- ✓ The PR interval should be constant

Sinus rhythm

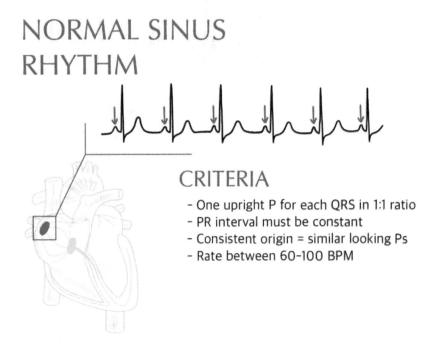

NORMAL SINUS RHYTHM

CRITERIA

- One upright P for each QRS in 1:1 ratio
- PR interval must be constant
- Consistent origin = similar looking Ps
- Rate between 60-100 BPM

What is normal sinus rhythm?

Sinus rhythm describes a cardiac impulse that begins in the SA node and follows the natural path of progression to the purkinje fibers in the ventricles.

What does this mean?

The term *normal*, indicates that the impulse is occurring at rate of 60 – 100 beats per minute, the inherent natural rate of discharge at the SA node.

Why should we care?

To understand deviations from normal, we first have to understand *what normal is*, or what it should be. Take home points are presented on the next page in the form of a rhythm cheat sheet and sample rhythm interpretation. We'll follow this format for the remaining rhythms throughout the book.

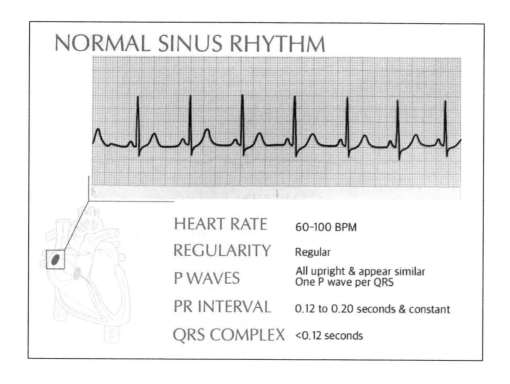

NORMAL SINUS RHYTHM

HEART RATE	60-100 BPM
REGULARITY	Regular
P WAVES	All upright & appear similar One P wave per QRS
PR INTERVAL	0.12 to 0.20 seconds & constant
QRS COMPLEX	<0.12 seconds

NORMAL SINUS RHYTHM

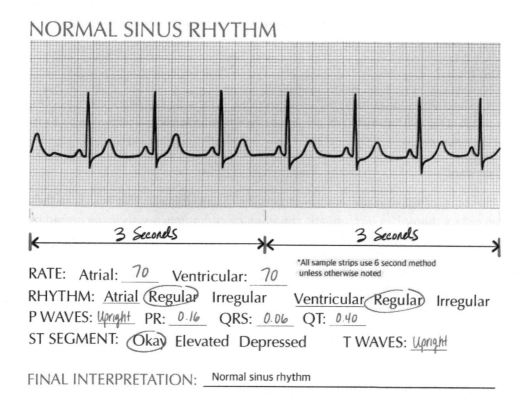

3 Seconds   3 Seconds

*All sample strips use 6 second method unless otherwise noted

RATE: Atrial: 70   Ventricular: 70

RHYTHM: Atrial (Regular) Irregular   Ventricular (Regular) Irregular

P WAVES: Upright   PR: 0.16   QRS: 0.06   QT: 0.40

ST SEGMENT: (Okay) Elevated Depressed   T WAVES: Upright

FINAL INTERPRETATION: Normal sinus rhythm

Follow along with the sample rhythm interpretation above using the concepts that we've discussed to this point. *Note that for all sample strips provided, we're using the 6 second strip method for heart rate evaluation unless otherwise noted.

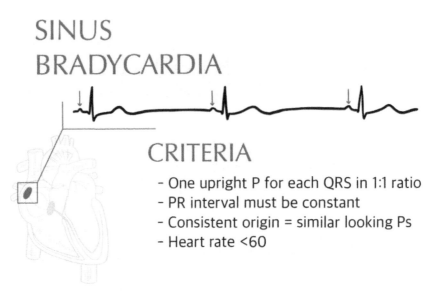

SINUS BRADYCARDIA

CRITERIA

- One upright P for each QRS in 1:1 ratio
- PR interval must be constant
- Consistent origin = similar looking Ps
- Heart rate <60

What is sinus bradycardia?

Sinus bradycardia (sinus = SA node, brady = slow, cardia = heart) describes a cardiac impulse that begins in the SA node and follows the natural path of progression to the purkinje fibers in the ventricles similar to normal sinus rhythm but at a slightly lower rate.

What does this mean?

Bradycardia is a descriptor indicating a rhythm slower than "normal" for the inherent pacemaker site, "sinus" in this case. This rhythm shares all the sinus rhythm criteria but specifically with a rate of less than 60 beats per minute.

Why should we care?

Patients in sinus bradycardia may present symptomatic or asymptomatic. This will guide the treatment of this rhythm or lack thereof. In fact, athletic conditioning commonly results in decreased resting heart rates. This is sometimes referred to as "Athlete's heart." Additional causes may include[17,24,25]:

- ✓ Medications (digoxin, beta blockers, and other AV nodal blocking agents including certain calcium channel blockers)
- ✓ Heart attacks, especially those affecting the right coronary artery which feeds the SA node
- ✓ Electrolyte imbalances
- ✓ Impaired coronary oxygen delivery due to atherosclerosis or coronary lesions
- ✓ During period of rest and sleep, enhanced vagal tones may slow the heart rate
- ✓ Increased intracranial pressure
- ✓ Hypoxia
- ✓ Hypothermia

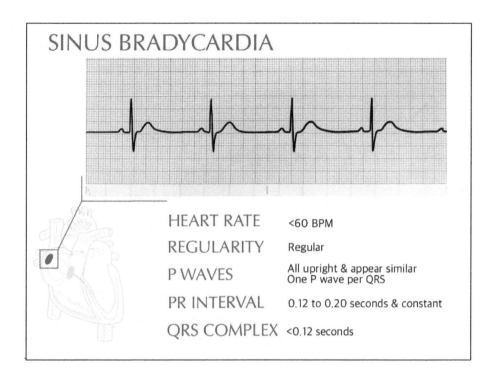

SINUS BRADYCARDIA

HEART RATE	<60 BPM
REGULARITY	Regular
P WAVES	All upright & appear similar One P wave per QRS
PR INTERVAL	0.12 to 0.20 seconds & constant
QRS COMPLEX	<0.12 seconds

SINUS BRADYCARDIA

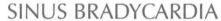
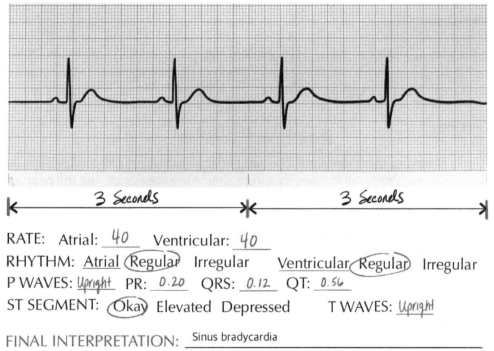

RATE: Atrial: 40   Ventricular: 40

RHYTHM: Atrial (Regular) Irregular   Ventricular (Regular) Irregular

P WAVES: Upright   PR: 0.20   QRS: 0.12   QT: 0.56

ST SEGMENT: (Okay) Elevated Depressed   T WAVES: Upright

FINAL INTERPRETATION: Sinus bradycardia

Follow along with the sample rhythm interpretation above using the concepts that we've discussed to this point.

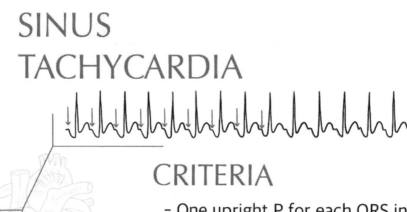

SINUS TACHYCARDIA

CRITERIA

- One upright P for each QRS in 1:1 ratio
- PR interval must be constant
- Consistent origin = similar looking Ps
- Heart rate >100

What is sinus tachycardia?

Sinus tachycardia (sinus = SA node, tachy = fast, cardia = heart) describes a cardiac impulse that begins in the SA node and follows the natural path of progression to the purkinje fibers in the ventricles similar to normal sinus rhythm but at a slightly faster rate.

What does this mean?

Sinus tachycardia maintains that there should be one upright P wave per QRS, the PR interval should remain constant with each cycle, all P waves should be similar in appearance, and the heart rate will be greater than 100 BPM.

Note that in the image above, there is a P wave preceding each QRS complex although they're partially buried within the usually smooth T wave of the preceding cardiac cycle. The main take away here is that they're coming on time every time and they're all similar in appearance. It's common at very high heart rates for the T wave to have a humped appearance at its peak. The humped T wave indicates the presence of P waves that are distorting the usually smooth deflection of the T wave.

Situation, along with the age-predicted maximum heart rate formula (AMPHR) may help provide additional insight[7,24]. Consider the acute care setting: is the patient out of bed and working with physical therapy while on telemetry, demonstrating a gradual rise in heart rate? If so, it may be sinus tachycardia. Are they resting comfortably in bed while experiencing a sudden spike in heart rate to 220 BPM? This would favor an arrhythmia of alternate origin.

Normal exercise induced sinus tachycardia rate maximums relative to patient age may provide additional situational information (220 – age = maximum predicted HR). For example, a 65-year-old individual would have a predicted sinus maximum of 155 BPM. Compare this to a 19-year-old individual with a predicted maximum of 201 BPM. Keep in mind, this formula only provides an estimation and is not without limitations.

Why should we care?

Treatment of sinus tachycardia should begin with assessment of the patient followed by treatment of the underlying cause. If they're in pain, can we help with the pain? If they're in distress, can we keep them calm while assessing for precipitating factors? If indicated, rate controlling medications such as beta blockers or calcium channel blockers may also play a role for patients that are chronically tachycardic[20].

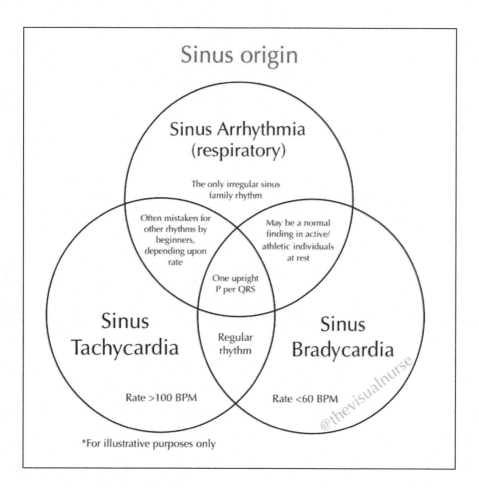

As a preface to the last sinus origin rhythm that we'll cover (sinus arrhythmia) here's a graphic comparing a few rhythms of sinus origin to help with differentiation.

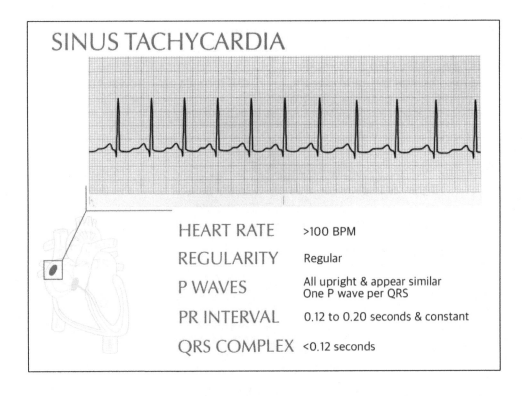

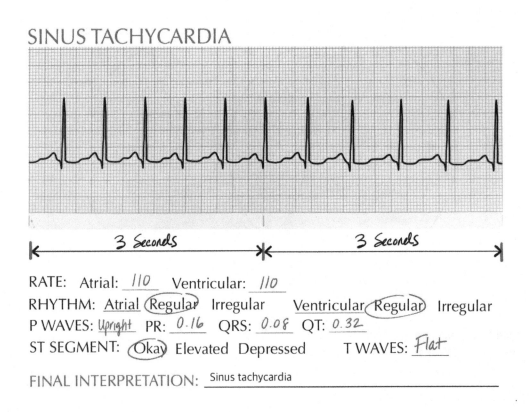

RATE: Atrial: _110_ Ventricular: _110_
RHYTHM: Atrial (Regular) Irregular   Ventricular (Regular) Irregular
P WAVES: _Upright_ PR: _0.16_ QRS: _0.08_ QT: _0.32_
ST SEGMENT: (Okay) Elevated Depressed   T WAVES: _Flat_

FINAL INTERPRETATION: _Sinus tachycardia_

Follow along with the sample rhythm interpretation above using the concepts that we've discussed to this point.

SINUS ARRHYTHMIA

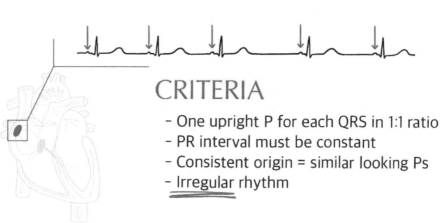

CRITERIA

- One upright P for each QRS in 1:1 ratio
- PR interval must be constant
- Consistent origin = similar looking Ps
- Irregular rhythm

What is sinus arrhythmia?

Two of the most common *irregularly* irregular rhythms are atrial fibrillation and sinus arrhythmia. There's one key difference. The P wave. Sinus arrhythmia is the major rhythm/arrhythmia of sinus origin that's irregular (excluding ectopic beats like premature atrial contractions).

What does this mean?

With *respiratory* sinus arrhythmia, the SA node discharges faster with inspiration and slower during exhalation creating an irregular rhythm. This is partly due to pressure changes in the thorax in addition to vagal tone modulation[25] and is a normal finding in healthy adults.

This variation has also been explained as representing a healthy balance between sympathetic and parasympathetic systems and is common in younger, active individuals. Loss of sinus rate variation with age suggests the healthy balance of autonomic systems may be affected and is even an early sign of heart disease[24].

Why should we care?

Don't confuse sinus arrhythmia with the other common irregular rhythm mentioned above. Like sinus arrhythmia, atrial fibrillation is irregular but this is not due to autonomic and/or pressure changes associated with ventilation. With atrial fibrillation, a lack of organized atrial contraction results in an unpredictable ventricular response. Comparatively, note the key characteristic of a 1:1 P wave to QRS complex ratio with sinus arrhythmia.

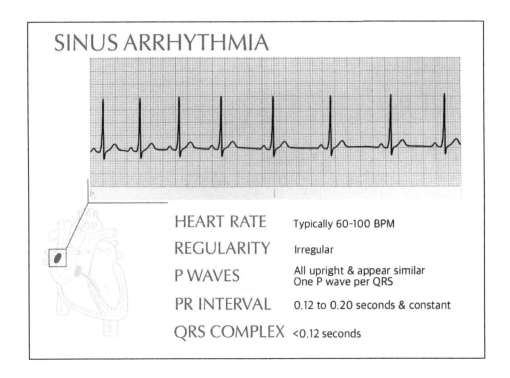

SINUS ARRHYTHMIA

HEART RATE	Typically 60-100 BPM
REGULARITY	Irregular
P WAVES	All upright & appear similar One P wave per QRS
PR INTERVAL	0.12 to 0.20 seconds & constant
QRS COMPLEX	<0.12 seconds

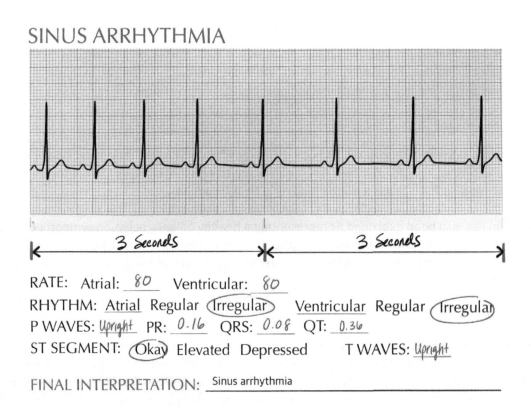

SINUS ARRHYTHMIA

3 Seconds   3 Seconds

RATE: Atrial: _80_   Ventricular: _80_

RHYTHM: Atrial Regular (Irregular)   Ventricular Regular (Irregular)

P WAVES: Upright   PR: 0.16   QRS: 0.08   QT: 0.36

ST SEGMENT: (Okay) Elevated Depressed   T WAVES: Upright

FINAL INTERPRETATION: _Sinus arrhythmia_

Follow along with the sample rhythm interpretation above using the concepts that we've discussed to this point.

ECG RATES
REFERENCE SHEET

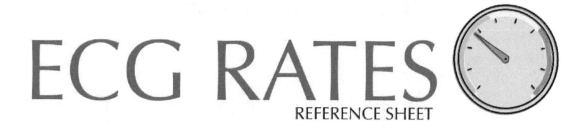

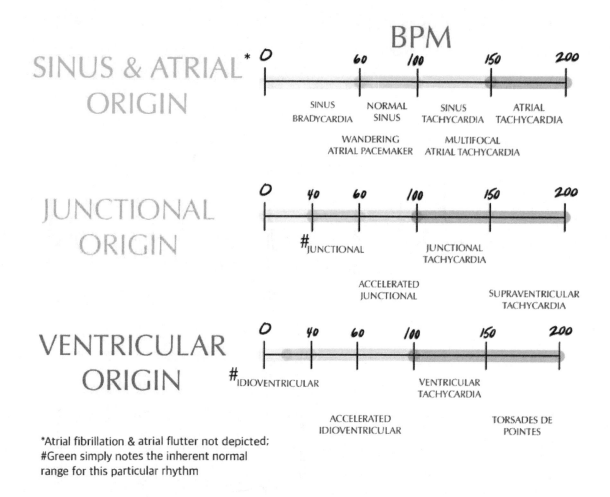

*Atrial fibrillation & atrial flutter not depicted;
#Green simply notes the inherent normal
range for this particular rhythm

This concludes the rhythms and arrhythmias of sinus origin. Next up we'll take a look at the arrhythmias of atrial origin (that are not necessarily sinus!) as we progress from top to bottom in our examination of potential cardiac conduction sites.

SINUS ORIGIN PRACTICE

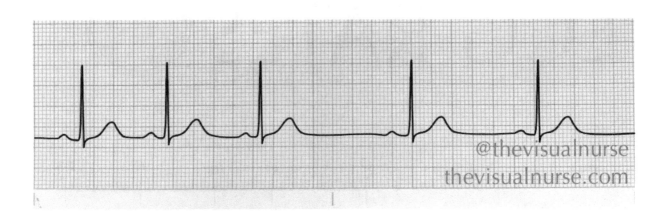

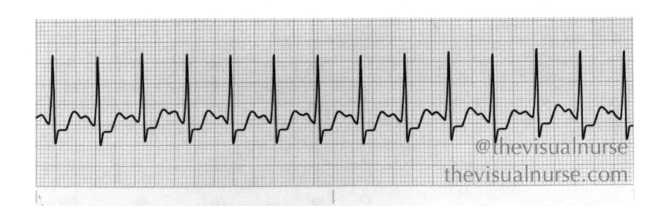

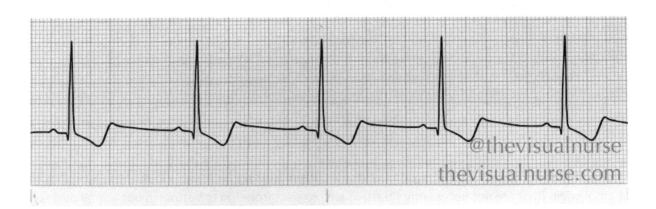

Turn to the "Rhythm strips answer key" section in the back of the book to check your answers!

CHAPTER 6: ARRHYTHMIAS OF ATRIAL ORIGIN... BUT NOT NECESSARILY SINUS!

ATRIAL TACHYCARDIA

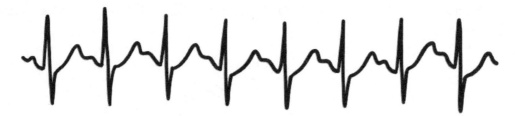

ATRIAL FLUTTER

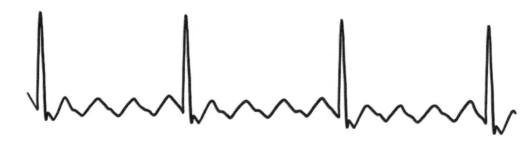

WANDERING ATRIAL

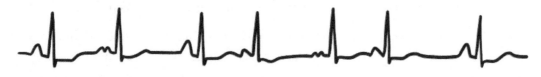

ATRIAL FIBRILLATION

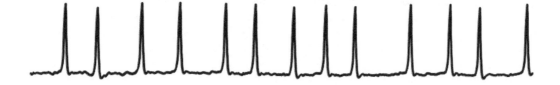

Following the rhythms and arrhythmias of sinus origin we progress to the arrhythmias of atrial origin.

What are atrial arrhythmias?

You may be thinking, "Aren't sinus and atrial similar?" And the answer is yes! ...almost.

What does this mean?

All sinus rhythms are atrial but not all atrial rhythms are sinus. This is because the SA node resides in the right atrium, but there's more to the atria than just the SA node. Think of it this way: the state of Wyoming (the square pictured below) is in the United States, but not all of the United States resides in the state of Wyoming.

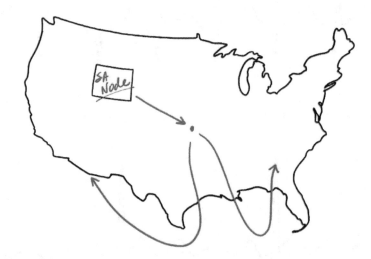

Why should we care?

Here are a few key points about atrial arrhythmias to help with differentiation and identification:

✓ Atrial arrhythmias originate from the atrial tissues but not necessarily the SA node (remember all cardiac cells possess some degree of automaticity under the right conditions and circumstances)
✓ Expect upright P waves/ atrial waves *except* for atrial fibrillation and some ectopic atrial rhythms
✓ If the P wave is inverted, look for a PR interval >0.12 seconds indicating longer atrial to ventricular travel time than for junctional origin rhythms
✓ The QRS should be narrow and less than 0.12 seconds in duration

Intro to ectopy: premature atrial contractions

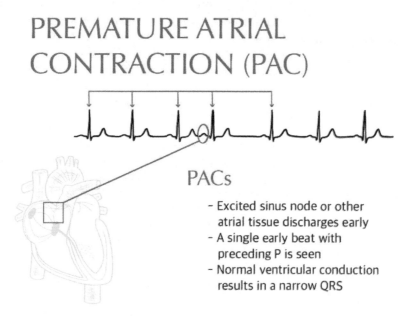

In the atrial origin category, we begin with an introduction to ectopic beats.

What are ectopic beats?

Ectopy is a word used to describe a (or multiple) cardiac conduction(s) that varies from the normal expected conduction pathway and timing, beginning with the SA node and terminating in the ventricles.

What does this mean?

Premature atrial contractions (PACs) are exactly what the name describes. They arrive prematurely, produce a single ectopic beat depicted as an upright P wave, and relay normal conduction to the ventricles (notice the QRS is still narrow following the PAC). Premature atrial beats may arise from an SA node that gets excited and fires early or may come from the surrounding atrial tissue.

If an early beat is coming from the atria, expect that it should still produce a *positive* (upright) P wave since the impulse is traveling toward the positive electrode (excluding inverted, normal PR P waves). This is the idea behind differentiating a premature atrial contraction from a premature junctional contraction (Chapter 7). For more on positive and negative deflections check out Chapter 2.

Premature atrial contractions have a few possible causes including excessive nicotine and stimulant use, infectious states, electrolyte imbalance, and perfusion defect, among others[17]. Quite commonly however, they occur without clear cause. Fortunately, they rarely require treatment unless they're really starting to cause symptoms (like palpitations). A cup of coffee or simply a sneeze may also cause isolated PACs. Not to worry.

Why should we care?

If symptomatic and any of the potential causes above can be isolated, treatment is usually aimed at correcting the underlying cause. If persistently symptomatic, a low dose rate controlling medication may be used to keep them under control. Once we understand the concept of atrial ectopic beats, we're ready to look at atrial arrhythmias. Let's go!

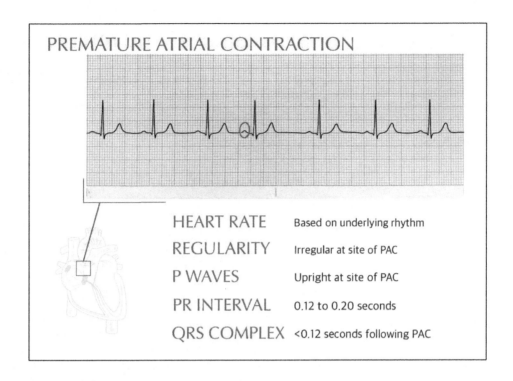

PREMATURE ATRIAL CONTRACTION

HEART RATE	Based on underlying rhythm
REGULARITY	Irregular at site of PAC
P WAVES	Upright at site of PAC
PR INTERVAL	0.12 to 0.20 seconds
QRS COMPLEX	<0.12 seconds following PAC

PREMATURE ATRIAL CONTRACTION

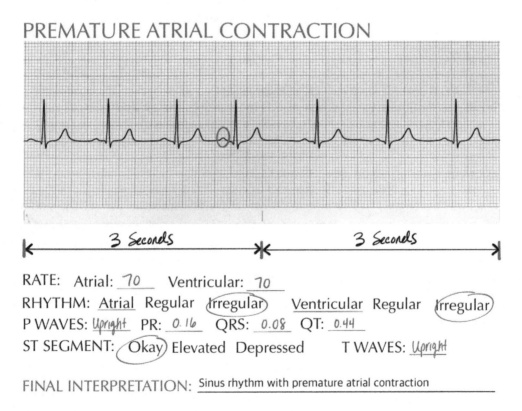

RATE: Atrial: _70_ Ventricular: _70_

RHYTHM: Atrial Regular (Irregular) Ventricular Regular (Irregular)

P WAVES: Upright PR: _0.16_ QRS: _0.08_ QT: _0.44_

ST SEGMENT: (Okay) Elevated Depressed T WAVES: Upright

FINAL INTERPRETATION: Sinus rhythm with premature atrial contraction

The sample rhythm strip above shows an underlying normal sinus rhythm with an isolated PAC.

✓ Note that the fourth beat that comes early, which is the PAC
✓ The underlying atrial and ventricular rhythm is regular when this early PAC is *ignored*

Wandering atrial pacemaker and multifocal atrial tachycardia

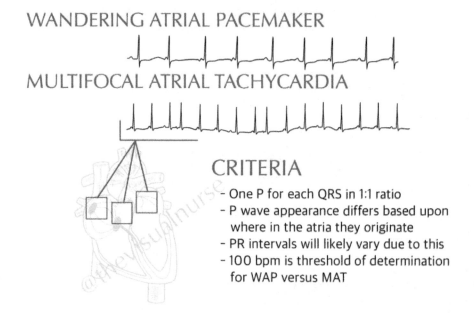

WANDERING ATRIAL PACEMAKER

MULTIFOCAL ATRIAL TACHYCARDIA

CRITERIA

- One P for each QRS in 1:1 ratio
- P wave appearance differs based upon where in the atria they originate
- PR intervals will likely vary due to this
- 100 bpm is threshold of determination for WAP versus MAT

For our purposes, think of these two rhythms as one in the same. The only difference? Heart rate. Is it above or below 100 beats per minute? If it's less than 100 BPM, you're looking at WAP. Greater than 100 BPM? You're looking at MAT[20].

What is a wandering atrial pacemaker?

The wandering atrial pacemaker has nothing to do with extrinsic cardiac hardware. The sino-atrial node is the *natural* pacemaker of the heart. Remember also that if P waves all appear similar and they're arriving at a rate of 60 – 100 beats per minute we *assume* them to be sinus. Why? My P waves may not look like your P waves. But if all my P waves look the same, they're said to have the same *morphology*. And if they have the same morphology, they're assumed to originate from the same site. But what if the morphology of the P wave is changing? Would that mean that it's coming from an alternate site?

Remember this example from chapter 3?

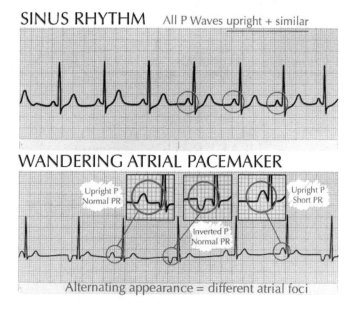

What does this mean?

This is exactly what happens in the case of the *wandering* atrial pacemaker. The pacemaker, the site is setting the pace for the rate of the heart, is *wandering* throughout the atria. This isn't entirely true... It's not travelling necessarily, but it describes a case in which there are multiple sites in the atria that are discharging and effectively *competing* to become the natural pacemaker. This results in at least three different P wave morphologies, a variable P – P interval, and often PR intervals that vary due to these alternate originations[25,26]. If the heart rate is less than 100 BPM we call this a wandering atrial pacemaker, or WAP. If it's greater than 100 BPM we call it a multifocal atrial tachycardia, or MAT for short.

Why should we care?

Causes of WAP and MAT might include lung diseases, oxygenation deficiencies, electrolyte abnormalities, stimulant use, drugs that mimic sympathetic nervous system effects[26] (like epinephrine) and others. Wandering atrial pacemaker is largely a benign rhythm. If the rate is too high (MAT), treating the underlying cause is typically the first step with rate controlling medications playing a role if needed. It's also worth noting that frequent premature atrial contractions on the ECG and/or multiple ectopic origins may precede atrial fibrillation[17] in part, due to increased atrial pressures and remodeling often seen in patients with lung diseases.

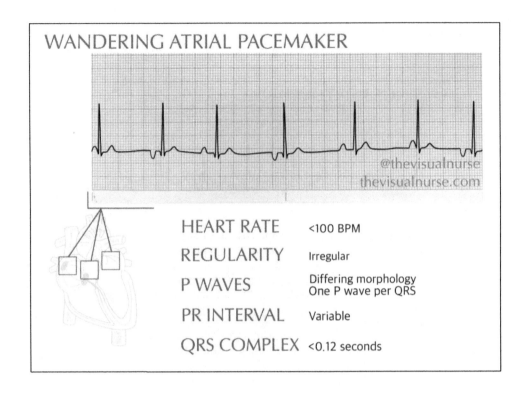

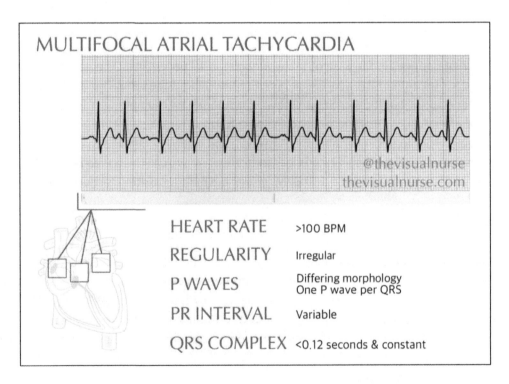

- ✓ Note that at very high rates MAT may mimic uncontrolled atrial fibrillation due to the irregular nature of the rhythm
- ✓ The key difference is the presence of P waves that are constantly changing in morphology. Compare with uncontrolled atrial fibrillation in the next section

WANDERING ATRIAL PACEMAKER

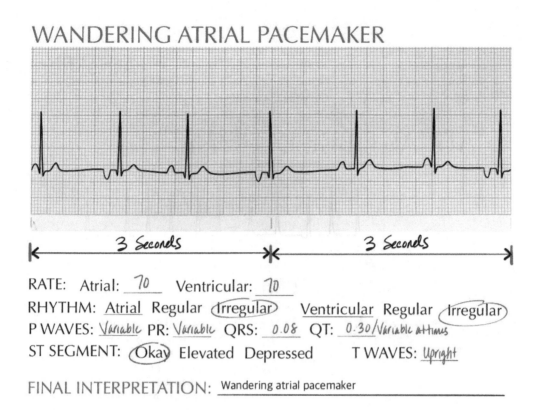

3 Seconds   3 Seconds

RATE: Atrial: _70_   Ventricular: _70_

RHYTHM: Atrial Regular (Irregular)   Ventricular Regular (Irregular)

P WAVES: _Variable_ PR: _Variable_ QRS: _0.08_ QT: _0.30/Variable at times_

ST SEGMENT: (Okay) Elevated Depressed   T WAVES: _Upright_

FINAL INTERPRETATION: _Wandering atrial pacemaker_

Follow along with the sample rhythm interpretation above using the concepts that we've discussed to this point.

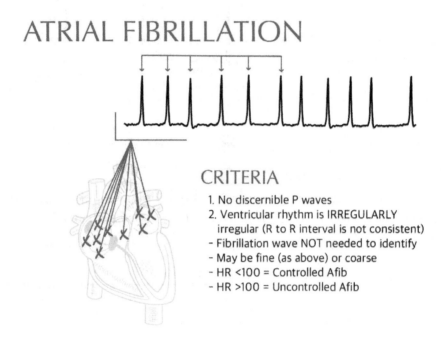

ATRIAL FIBRILLATION

CRITERIA

1. No discernible P waves
2. Ventricular rhythm is IRREGULARLY
   irregular (R to R interval is not consistent)
- Fibrillation wave NOT needed to identify
- May be fine (as above) or coarse
- HR <100 = Controlled Afib
- HR >100 = Uncontrolled Afib

What is atrial fibrillation?

Atrial fibrillation is characterized by chaotic and completely disorganized atrial depolarization. In fact, the atria are initiating between 300 – 600 beats each minute[27]!

What does this mean?

The atria are unable to coordinate adequate contractions. Because of this, blood tends to pool in the upper chambers and creates a favorable environment for the formation of clots. With a lack of coordinated atrial activity, the ventricles respond sporadically to the impulses being passed down from above. The result is an unpredictable and *irregularly irregular* ventricular response. Atrial impulses are conducted through the AV to the ventricles resulting in a narrow QRS (excluding aberrant conduction)., By doing so, the AV node plays a protective role by not allowing the ventricles to attempt to keep pace with the 300 + atrial impulses each minute[24].

On your rhythm strip, the two most important characteristics in recognizing atrial fibrillation are:

- ✓ **A rhythm that is *irregularly* irregular**
- ✓ **No discernible P waves present**

Compare this to MAT in the previous section in which the rhythm is irregular, but P waves are present with differing appearances. When evaluating a rhythm strip, if you notice a rhythm that is irregularly irregular and you find yourself having to justify whether or not P waves are present, chances are that you're looking at atrial fibrillation. At heart rates approaching 180 – 200 BPM and above, it may be increasingly difficult to determine the irregularity of the rhythm strip[27], in which case a pair of calipers will come in handy.

Ventricular response is a special concern in atrial fibrillation. With cardiac output already potentially impaired due to the underperforming atria, very rapid heart rates may further decrease cardiac output due to decreases in diastolic ventricular filling times and irregularly occurring ventricular beats[28]. At high heart rates, these patients may be prone to symptoms of fatigue, dizziness, imbalance, and more. Rate control is imperative in these cases.

Why should we care?

Atrial fibrillation is the most common sustained arrhythmia in the general population[28] with approximately 33% of arrhythmia related hospitalizations being attributed to A-fib[27]. Expect to encounter it at some point. Additionally, the "atrial kick" that sends blood forward to the ventricles is responsible for an estimated 10-30% of total cardiac output. Therefore, patients with atrial fibrillation may potentially experience meaningful decreases in total cardiac output which may worsen with very rapid heart rates. Treatment goals for atrial fibrillation include stroke prevention, rate control, and rhythm control.

A note on atrial fibrillation:

1. If the rhythm is *irregularly* irregular &

2. You have to convince yourself that you're seeing P waves

It's probably* A-fib

instagram: @thevisualnurse
www.thevisualnurse.com

———— The Visual Nurse ————

---

*Differentials may include WAP, MAT, and more.

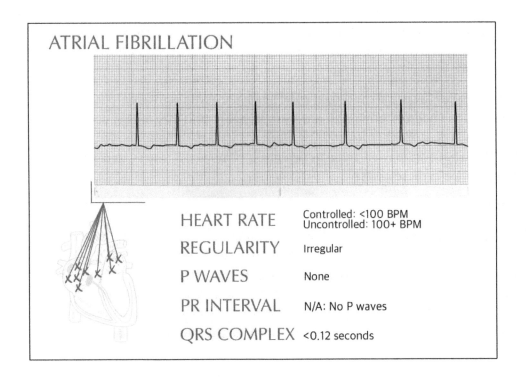

ATRIAL FIBRILLATION

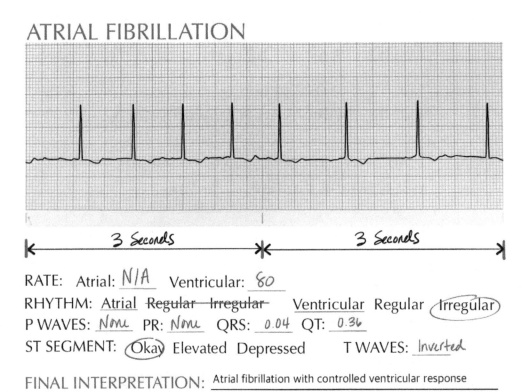

RATE: Atrial: N/A   Ventricular: 80

RHYTHM: Atrial ~~Regular~~ ~~Irregular~~   Ventricular Regular (Irregular)

P WAVES: None PR: None QRS: 0.04 QT: 0.36

ST SEGMENT: (Okay) Elevated Depressed   T WAVES: Inverted

FINAL INTERPRETATION: Atrial fibrillation with controlled ventricular response

Follow along with the sample rhythm interpretation above using the concepts that we've discussed to this point.

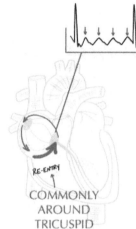

ATRIAL FLUTTER

CRITERIA

- Flutter waves should outnumber QRS
- Atrial rhythm regular due to circuit re-entry (left)
- Ventricular conduction ratio will determine regularity or irregularity (2:1, 3:1, 4:1, 5:1, or variable)

RE-ENTRY

COMMONLY AROUND TRICUSPID

What is atrial flutter?

Atrial flutter is typically presented on rhythm exams with the classic *sawtooth appearance*, describing the formation of the flutter (atrial) waves; they resemble the teeth on a saw. This is commonly a result of a singular impulse feeding back into itself at a very rapid rate. Note that flutter waves may have a positive or negative deflection, particularly in the limb leads, depending on if the impulse is travelling clockwise or counterclockwise, or is originating in the left versus right atrium[20]. The sawtooth appearance isn't always as easy to depict as it may seem.

What does this mean?

Flutter waves largely outnumber the QRS complexes and thankfully they do. These flutter waves commonly occur in the ballpark of 250 to 350 per minute[19,20,24]. Like our atrial fibrillation scenario, could you imagine what would happen if the ventricles were responded to each flutter wave? A 1:1 ratio would mean a ventricular rate around 300 BPM more or less; something not likely compatible with life long-term due to the whole *"cardiac output increases with rate until it has a negative effect on ventricular filling time,"* thing we discussed earlier. Remember also what we said about the concept of ventricular refractoriness back in Chapter 3.

On the rhythm strip, atrial flutter should be characterized by:

- ✓ More flutter waves than QRS complexes (except in 1:1 conduction)
- ✓ An atrial rhythm that is relatively regular and predictable in the 200 -300 beat per minute range
- ✓ Ventricular response may be variable, which means it may be regular OR irregular
- ✓ Ventricular conduction may commonly range from 2:1 to 5:1 or higher, atrial:ventricular

The conduction ratio may not always be consistent. It's possible to have a QRS every second atrial beat followed by four atrial beats before the next QRS. It can be a mixed bag of sorts. This would be an example of an *irregularly irregular* rhythm, a lack of predictable pattern. Atrial flutter has the capability to present in any of the three rhythm *regularity* possibilities.

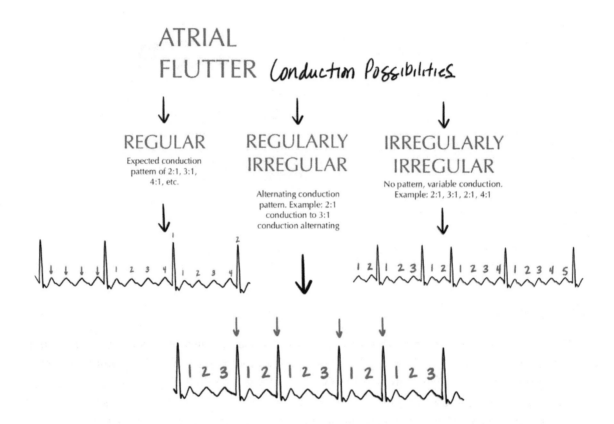

Why should we care?

Atrial flutter typically results from an abnormal conduction pathway feeding back into and activating itself repeatedly (macro-reentry). The result is way more flutter waves than QRS with the QRS essentially responding where they can. Causes of atrial flutter may include structural heart disease, sepsis, heart attack, atrial surgeries, and scar tissue formation, and more[20]. It may also be idiopathic. Treatment for these patients is typically aimed at rate and rhythm control and may include ablation to burn out the area of the faulty circuit if the arrhythmia persists beyond conservative treatment attempts.

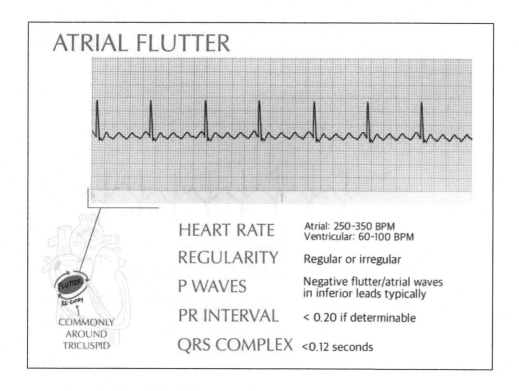

ATRIAL FLUTTER

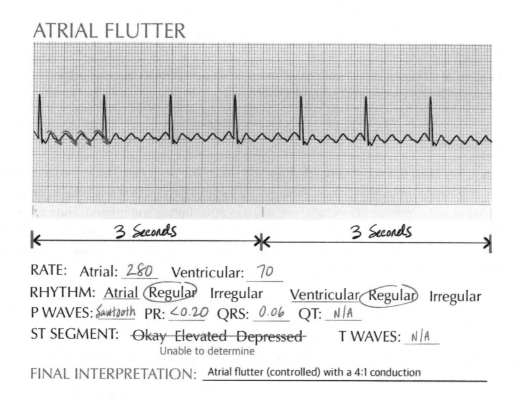

RATE: Atrial: 280 Ventricular: 70

RHYTHM: Atrial (Regular) Irregular   Ventricular (Regular) Irregular

P WAVES: Sawtooth PR: <0.20 QRS: 0.06 QT: N/A

ST SEGMENT: ~~Okay Elevated Depressed~~   T WAVES: N/A
Unable to determine

FINAL INTERPRETATION: Atrial flutter (controlled) with a 4:1 conduction

Follow along with the sample rhythm interpretation above using the concepts that we've discussed to this point, but be aware of the following:

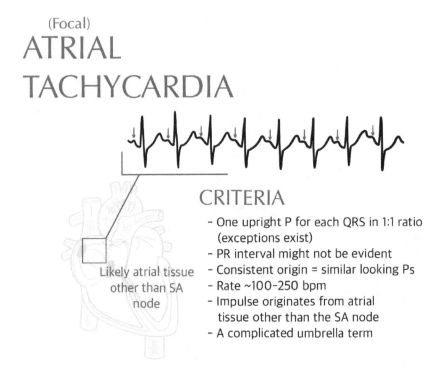

(Focal)
ATRIAL TACHYCARDIA

Likely atrial tissue
other than SA
node

CRITERIA

- One upright P for each QRS in 1:1 ratio (exceptions exist)
- PR interval might not be evident
- Consistent origin = similar looking Ps
- Rate ~100-250 bpm
- Impulse originates from atrial tissue other than the SA node
- A complicated umbrella term

What is atrial tachycardia?

Not suprisingly, atrial tachycardia falls under the umbrella of 'arrhythmias of atrial origin'. It also falls under the supraventricular tachycardia umbrella. We'll take a look at why when we dig into SVT in Chapter 7.

What does this mean?

All sinus rhythms are atrial but not all atrial rhythms are sinus. The term *atrial* tachycardia indicates that the impulse is originating from atrial tissue, although we can't be certain that it is sinus in origin. Two major categories of atrial tachycardia include: reentry (i.e. atrial flutter and others), and ectopic/focal atrial site. Some sources will differentiate sinus tachycardia from atrial tachycardia using a rate of 150 BPM as a threshold[17]. Around this rate, the T and P waves often slur together making if difficult to measure the PR and QT intervals.

You can see why "atrial tachycardia" is one of my least favorite arrhythmia distinctions. In my opinion, what's far more important is what the patient was doing before the heart rate reached ~150 BPM. Were they exercising with a gradual rate increase? If so, it's more likely sinus tachycardia. Were they resting comfortably before the rate spiked quickly into this range? If so, may be some form of atrial tachycardia[24] (ectopic/focal atrial).

We should mention here that atrial P waves can sometimes be inverted. In this case, the PR interval is the key because it tells us about the travel time to the AV node and ventricles. If the P is inverted with a normal PR interval, it's taking a longer time to reach the ventricles than a junctional P wave would and indicates a likely atrial origin. In this case we'd refer to this as an *atrial ectopic rhythm if <100 BPM* and an *atrial tachycardia if >100 BPM*.

Why should we care?

Atrial tachycardia is technically a form of supraventricular tachycardia, although one of the less common forms. Understanding this arrhythmia now will help with our understanding of SVT in later chapters. The key here is the presence of P/atrial waves with a rate *likely* ~100-250 BPM[17] although wider ranges are observed[20]. In the examples that follow, note the appearance of a double humped T wave in the rhythm strip. This distortion is due to the presence of regularly recurring P waves.

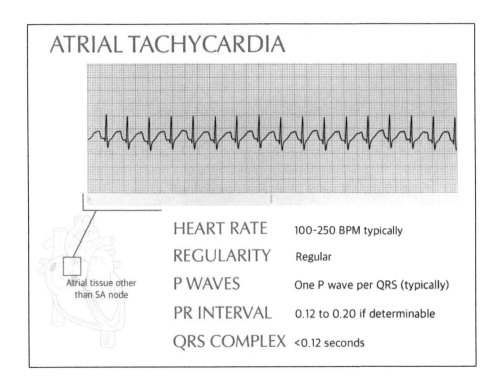

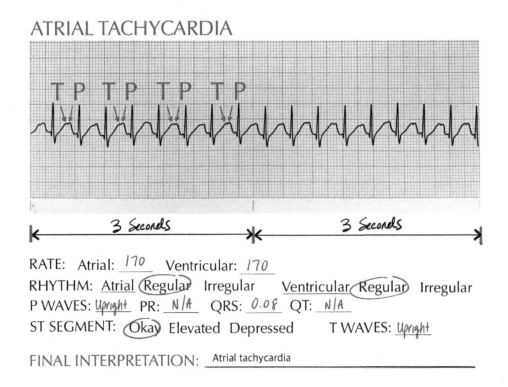

Follow along with the sample rhythm interpretation above using the concepts that we've discussed to this point. Note the "double humped" T waves indicate the presence of a regularly recurring P/atrial wave buried within.

ECG RATES

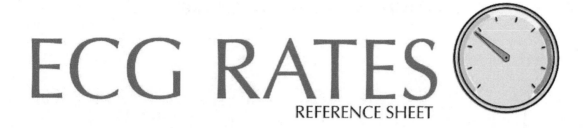

REFERENCE SHEET

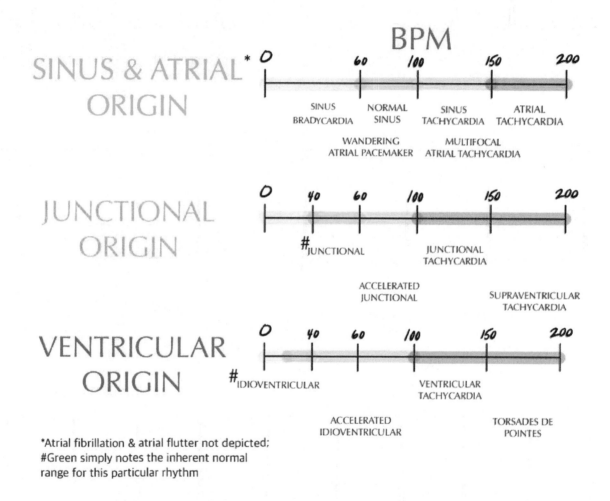

*Atrial fibrillation & atrial flutter not depicted;
#Green simply notes the inherent normal
range for this particular rhythm

This concludes the arrhythmias of atrial origin. Next up we'll take a look at rhythms and arrhythmias of junctional origin as we progress from top to bottom in our examination of potential cardiac conduction sites.

ATRIAL ORIGIN PRACTICE

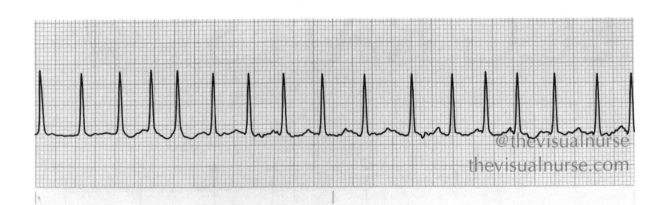

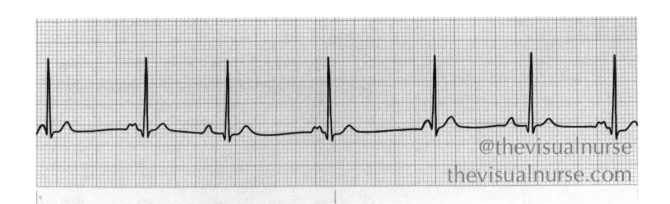

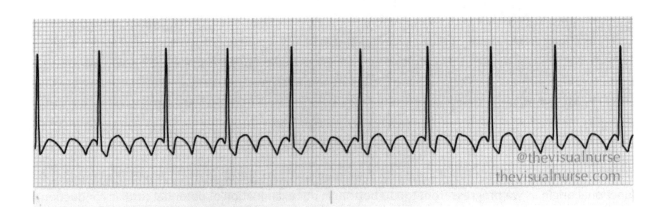

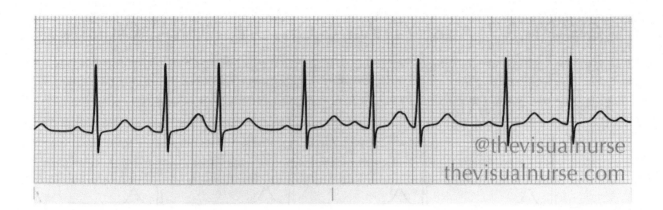

Turn to the "Rhythm strips answer key" section in the back of the book to check your answers!

CHAPTER 7: ARRHYTHMIAS OF JUNCTIONAL ORIGIN

JUNCTIONAL

ACCELERATED
JUNCTIONAL

JUNCTIONAL
TACHYCARDIA

SUPRAVENTRICULAR
TACHYCARDIA

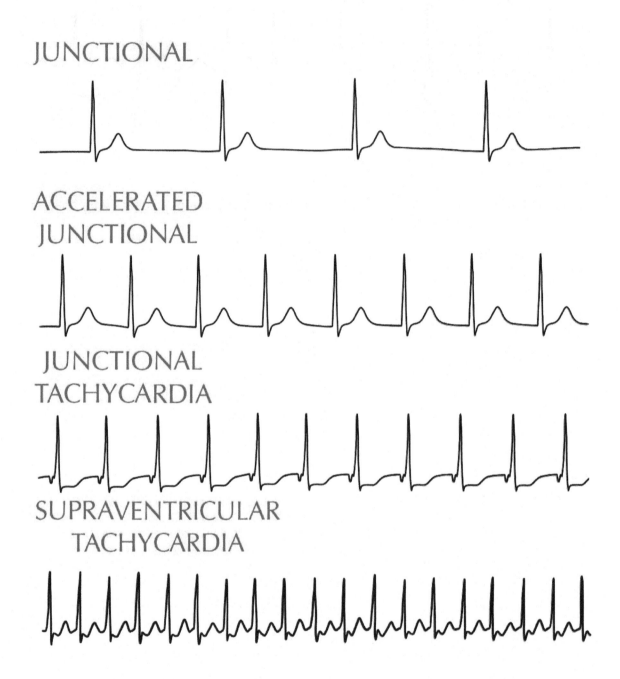

JUNCTIONAL RHYTHMS

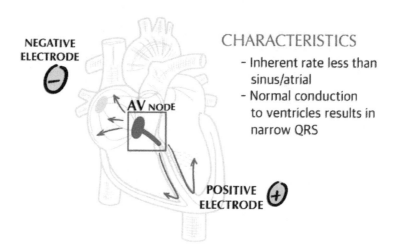

NEGATIVE ELECTRODE

$\ominus$

AV NODE

POSITIVE ELECTRODE $\oplus$

CHARACTERISTICS

- Inherent rate less than sinus/atrial
- Normal conduction to ventricles results in narrow QRS

What comes to mind when you hear the term "junctional?" Where is the AV junction located? How does this affect the ECG?

What is a junctional rhythm?

If the sinus pacemaker fails, the next in line *should* take over as the new pacemaker of the heart. After the sinus and atrial mechanisms, the AV *junction* is the next downstream to pick up responsibilities of pacing the heart. The AV *bundle* (aka bundle of His) permits electrical conduction across the insulation between the atria and ventricles. This communication is regulated by the AV *node*[24]. We'll examine this site as we follow the natural progression of the depolarization pathway.

What does this mean?

The pacemaker cells surrounding the AV junction can initiate regular impulses but at a slightly lower natural rate than their sinus and atrial superiors[11]. The heart is built this way so that when the pacemaker cells with the fastest intrinsic rate are in action, those below with slower intrinsic rates are suppressed and function primarily to pass along the impulse from above.

When the impulse starts at the AV junction, the upper atria may depolarize in *retrograde*, meaning in reverse from the natural depolarization pathway. This makes sense since the AV junction is downstream and must feed the impulse back upstream to the upper chambers, traveling *away from* the positive electrode. (For a review on positive and negative ECG deflections review see Chapter 2.) Each impulse is also conducted *normally,* down to the ventricles. Therefore, we expect to see a narrow QRS with junctional rhythms.

Why should we care?

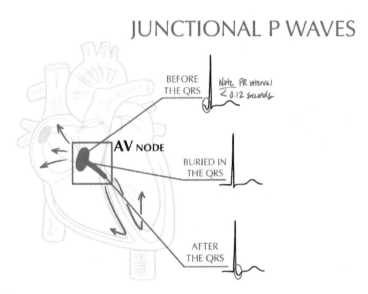

P waves associated with junctional rhythms have three potential appearances: inverted before the QRS, buried within the QRS, or inverted after the QRS[24]. The appearance will depend on how high or low the impulse is located along the conduction pathway.

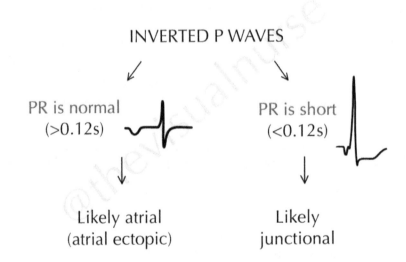

The sinus node typically outpaces other inferior pacemaker sites within the heart[11]. Junctional origin rates are inherently slower, and ventricular origin rates are even slower than junctional. To properly identify junctional rhythms, we need to have a firm grasp on identifying both P waves as well as heart rates.

RHYTHMS OF JUNCTIONAL ORIGIN

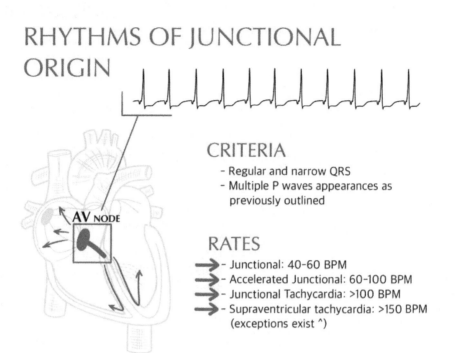

CRITERIA

- Regular and narrow QRS
- Multiple P waves appearances as previously outlined

RATES

- Junctional: 40-60 BPM
- Accelerated Junctional: 60-100 BPM
- Junctional Tachycardia: >100 BPM
- Supraventricular tachycardia: >150 BPM (exceptions exist ^)

The criteria assigned to junctional rhythms are listed above along with associated rates for each. Be advised that some sources depict inherent junctional rates around 25 – 40 BPM and accelerated values above 50 BPM[24]. For our purposes and for clean consistency across many nursing texts we'll be referencing the values in the image above[22]. Alright, enough overview. Let's look at some examples!

Junctional rhythm

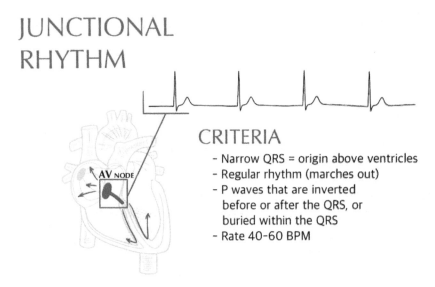

JUNCTIONAL RHYTHM

CRITERIA
- Narrow QRS = origin above ventricles
- Regular rhythm (marches out)
- P waves that are inverted before or after the QRS, or buried within the QRS
- Rate 40-60 BPM

What is a normal junctional rhythm?

First up is the normal junctional rhythm, also called junctional *escape* rhythm. I like to think of escape rhythms as those that take over as a fail-safe if upstream sites fail[24] (an oversimplified explanation). In this case, it helps me remember that 40 BPM is the (relative) upper limit for the inherent junctional range. Compare this to accelerated and junctional tachycardia in the ensuing sections. Notice the key characteristics of an inverted or absent P wave and a rate between 40 and 60 BPM.

What does this mean?

This rhythm represents the natural depolarization rate for the AV junction. The key is to first notice the rate and regularity of the rhythm. Junctional rhythms should march out regularly, letting you know the impulse is coming from a dependable pacemaker (as opposed to atrial fibrillation). The next characteristic to notice is the narrow QRS. A narrow QRS indicates to us that the impulse is *supraventricular* in origin, meaning that it originates *above* the ventricles. Altogether with a regular rhythm coming 40 – 60 times per minute, inverted or absent P waves, and a narrow QRS, the interpretation of a junctional rhythm can be made.

Why should we care?

This rhythm may be idiopathic and benign. In fact, healthy individuals may present with this rhythm at rest or while sleeping. Other potential causes may include heart attacks (especially with right coronary artery involvement), AV nodal blocking agents/medications, and sick sinus nodes, among others[17]. Assess your patient for precipitating contributors, symptoms associated with bradycardia, and notify the provider as needed.

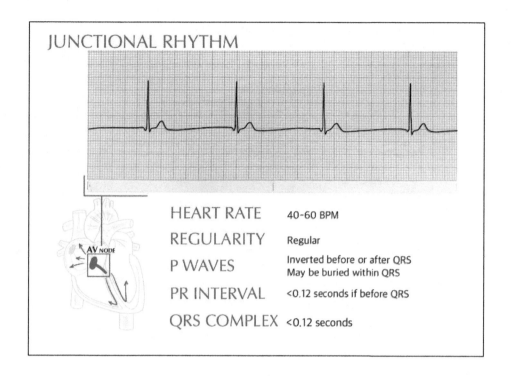

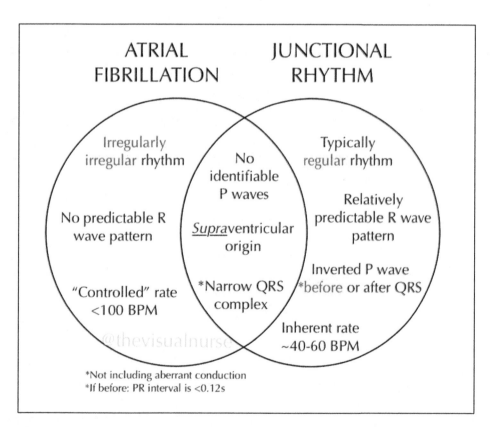

Junctional rhythms and atrial fibrillation can be tough to differentiate, especially in cases of very fine atrial fibrillation where the atrial baseline is very near iso-electric. Forget using fibrillation waves as part of your criteria for this reason and check out the graphic above. The regularity may be the key. Exceptions exist (i.e. atrial fibrillation with presence of complete heart block)

JUNCTIONAL RHYTHM

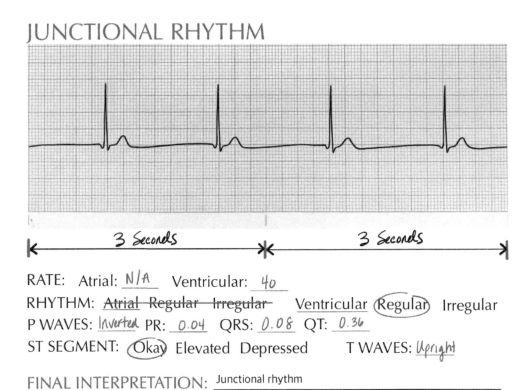

RATE: Atrial: N/A   Ventricular: 40

RHYTHM: ~~Atrial Regular Irregular~~   Ventricular (Regular) Irregular

P WAVES: Inverted   PR: 0.04   QRS: 0.08   QT: 0.36

ST SEGMENT: (Okay) Elevated Depressed   T WAVES: Upright

FINAL INTERPRETATION: Junctional rhythm

Follow along with the sample rhythm interpretation above using the concepts that we've discussed to this point.

✓ Are the atria depolarizing with each beat seen above? Yes, but in retrograde as we discussed which means they're activated by the AV junction. Notice the inverted P wave just before the QRS complex

✓ This is why the P wave is inverted. Since there is no sinus or atrial *initiation* of impulse, we list the atrial rate as not applicable

Accelerated junctional rhythm

ACCELERATED JUNCTIONAL

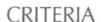

CRITERIA

- Narrow QRS = origin above ventricles
- Regular rhythm (marches out)
- P waves that are inverted
  before or after the QRS, or
  buried within the QRS
- Rate 60-100 BPM

AV NODE

What is an accelerated junctional rhythm?

In the junctional origin category, think of the accelerated junctional rhythm as the older sibling to the normal junctional rhythm.

What does this mean?

When you examine this rhythm, you'll notice that the criteria remain the same throughout. The difference lies in the heart rate. You should still find a relatively regular rhythm with no upright P waves and a narrow QRS. Rather than the inherent junctional depolarization rate of 40 – 60 BPM, expect a rate between 60 and 100 BPM which is slightly accelerated.

Why should we care?

The key to rhythm identification begins with understanding inherent rates for each pacemaker site and moving up the scale from there to assess if a rhythm is accelerated or tachycardic (sinus: 60 – 100 BPM; junctional: 40 – 60 BPM; ventricular: 20 – 40 BPM). Assess your patient and notify the provider of changes from baseline. Causes of accelerated and tachycardic junctional rhythms may include diseases of the SA node, electrolyte imbalance, heart disease, cardiac glycoside toxicity (digitalis), and hypoxemia[17,24].

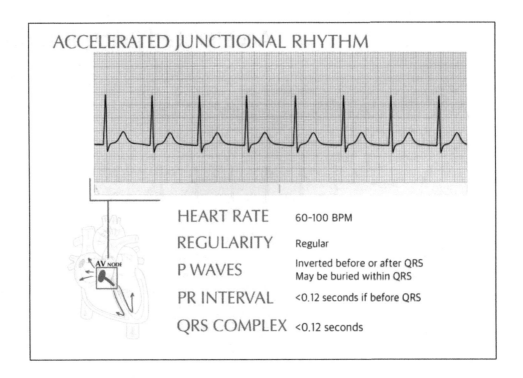

ACCELERATED JUNCTIONAL RHYTHM

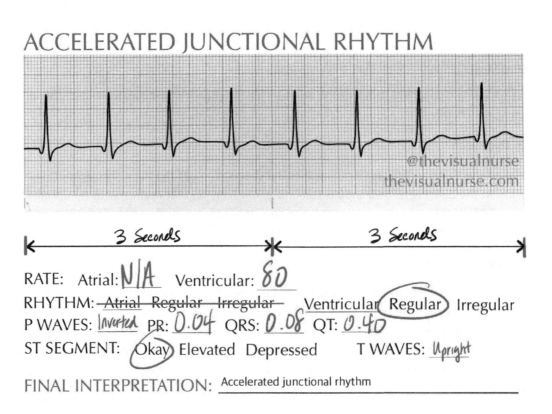

@thevisualnurse
thevisualnurse.com

|← 3 Seconds →|← 3 Seconds →|

RATE: Atrial: N/A   Ventricular: 80

RHYTHM: ~~Atrial   Regular   Irregular~~   Ventricular (Regular) Irregular

P WAVES: Inverted   PR: 0.04   QRS: 0.08   QT: 0.40

ST SEGMENT: (Okay) Elevated Depressed   T WAVES: Upright

FINAL INTERPRETATION: Accelerated junctional rhythm

Follow along with the sample rhythm interpretation above using the concepts that we've discussed to this point.

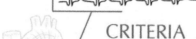

JUNCTIONAL
TACHYCARDIA

CRITERIA

- Narrow QRS = origin above ventricles
- Regular rhythm (marches out)
- P waves that are inverted
  before or after the QRS, or
  buried within the QRS
- Rate >100 BPM

AV NODE

What is junctional tachycardia?

If accelerated junctional is the big brother, then junctional tachycardia is the oldest sibling here (sometimes referred to as junctional ectopic tachycardia, or JET).

What does this mean?

All prior criteria for junctional rhythms remain but at a rate >100 BPM[22].

Why should we care?

At higher rates, this rhythm might mimic atrial fibrillation with a rapid ventricular response (AF-RVR). As heart rate increases and with a lack of discernible P waves it may become difficult to tell whether the rhythm is regular or irregular. A pair of calipers will come in handy in these cases to make the call but often, observing a continual rhythm strip for a longer period will inevitably offer subtle clues to the irregularity in A-fib as the QRS complexes dance closer to and further from one another. At this point, we've mentioned three rhythms that are very close in appearance at higher heart rates but can be differentiated using careful observation.

IRREGULAR WITH P WAVES

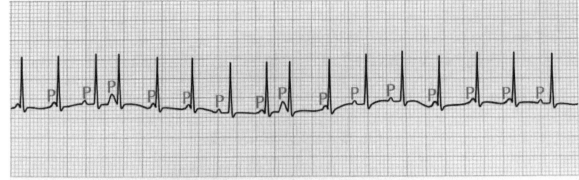

IRREGULAR, NO P WAVES

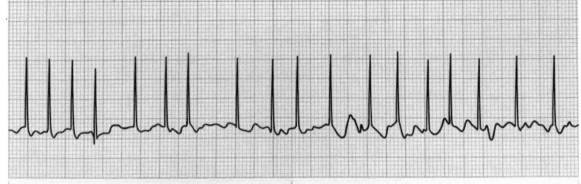

REGULAR, NO P WAVES

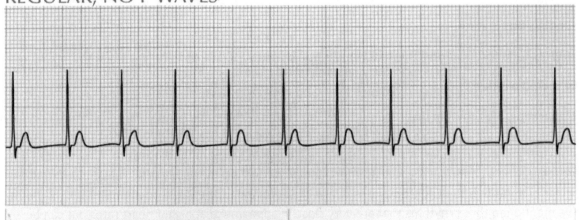

From top to bottom:

- ✓ Multifocal atrial tachycardia: P waves with alternating appearance, *irregular* rhythm
- ✓ Rapid atrial fibrillation: No discernible P waves, *irregular* rhythm
- ✓ Junctional tachycardia: Inverted or absent P waves, *regular* rhythm

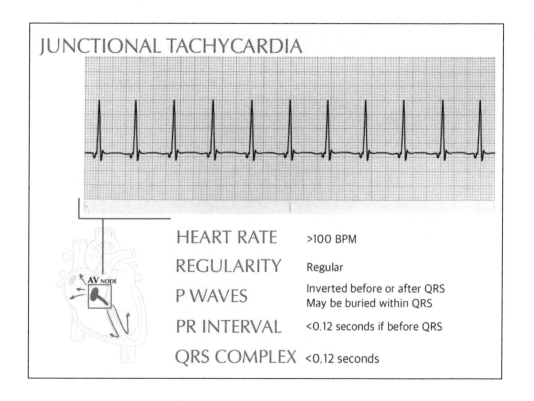

JUNCTIONAL TACHYCARDIA

HEART RATE	>100 BPM
REGULARITY	Regular
P WAVES	Inverted before or after QRS May be buried within QRS
PR INTERVAL	<0.12 seconds if before QRS
QRS COMPLEX	<0.12 seconds

JUNCTIONAL TACHYCARDIA

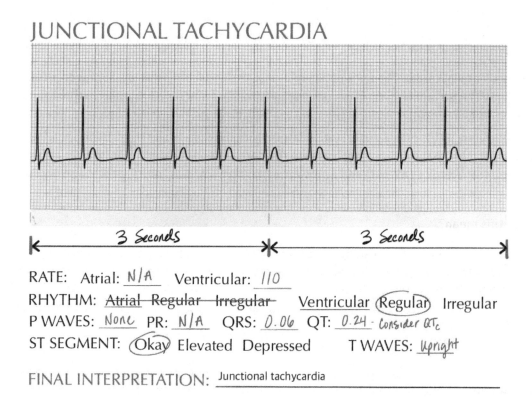

3 Seconds | 3 Seconds

RATE: Atrial: N/A Ventricular: 110
RHYTHM: ~~Atrial Regular Irregular~~ Ventricular (Regular) Irregular
P WAVES: None PR: N/A QRS: 0.06 QT: 0.24 - Consider QT$_c$
ST SEGMENT: (Okay) Elevated Depressed   T WAVES: Upright

FINAL INTERPRETATION: Junctional tachycardia

Follow along with the sample rhythm interpretation above using the concepts that we've discussed to this point.

Supraventricular tachycardia: a category in itself

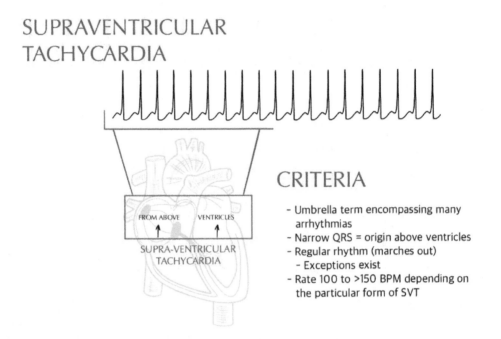

SUPRAVENTRICULAR
TACHYCARDIA

FROM ABOVE   VENTRICLES

SUPRA-VENTRICULAR
TACHYCARDIA

CRITERIA

- Umbrella term encompassing many arrhythmias
- Narrow QRS = origin above ventricles
- Regular rhythm (marches out)
  - Exceptions exist
- Rate 100 to >150 BPM depending on the particular form of SVT

What is supraventricular tachycardia?

Supraventricular tachycardia. The apex of all junctional and atrial arrhythmias. Supraventricular tachycardia (SVT) is an umbrella term encompassing atrial and junctional rhythms originating *above* the ventricles (SUPRA-ventricular), particularly from the bundle of His or above[20]. This includes inappropriate sinus tachycardias, focal and macro-reentry (flutter) atrial tachycardias, junctional tachycardias, and to what most nursing texts are referring when they use the term SVT: atrioventricular nodal reentry tachycardias (AVNRT) and atrioventricular tachycardias (AVRT; utilizing an accessory A to V pathway)[29].

What does this mean?

For this reason, rates may fall into an extremely broad range exceeding 100 to 250 BPM or greater depending upon the arrhythmia of interest. The hallmark of SVT in most nursing programs is a rapid narrow complex QRS with no identifiable P waves (with exception) at a rate greater than 150 BPM but this is largely an arbitrary number. The rhythm is typically regular... although there are exceptions.

Why should we care?

Let's be clear: many writings and exams are going to picture a *regular* rhythm like the one shown above. They'll show you a rhythm like the ones in the examples that follow at a rate >150 BPM. Just know that you're smarter than the average student or new nurse. You understand that in reality, SVT is the term used to describe many tachycardias (>100 BPM) originating above the ventricles, whether regular *or* irregular.

Classically though, when we use the term SVT, we're commonly referring to AV nodal re-entry tachycardias (AVNRT) or atrioventricular re-entry tachycardias (AVRT). A more appropriate term you may see is *Paroxysmal SVT (PSVT),* a subset of the "SVT umbrella". As outlined in the guidelines set forth by the American College of Cardiology, American Heart Association, and Heart Rhythm Society, PSVT is denoting a regular and rapid tachycardia with abrupt initiation and termination[20,29]. Keep in mind that AVNRT and AVRT can be sustained and may be stable or unstable (producing signs and symptoms of hemodynamic compromise). Paroxysmal SVT has quite a wide rate range, from around 100 to 250 BPM or greater.

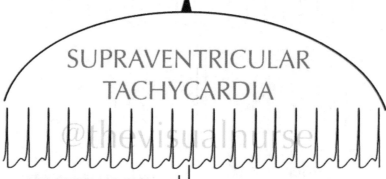

SUPRAVENTRICULAR TACHYCARDIA

PAROXYSMAL SVT
(PSVT/AVNRT/AVRT)

RAPID ATRIAL FLUTTER

RAPID ATRIAL FIBRILLATION

MULTIFOCAL ATRIAL TACHYCARDIA

FOCAL ATRIAL TACHYCARDIA

JUNCTIONAL TACHYCARDIA

CRITERIA

- *Narrow QRS
- Rates range >100 to 250+ based on type
- Origin above ventricles

*Excludes aberrant conduction

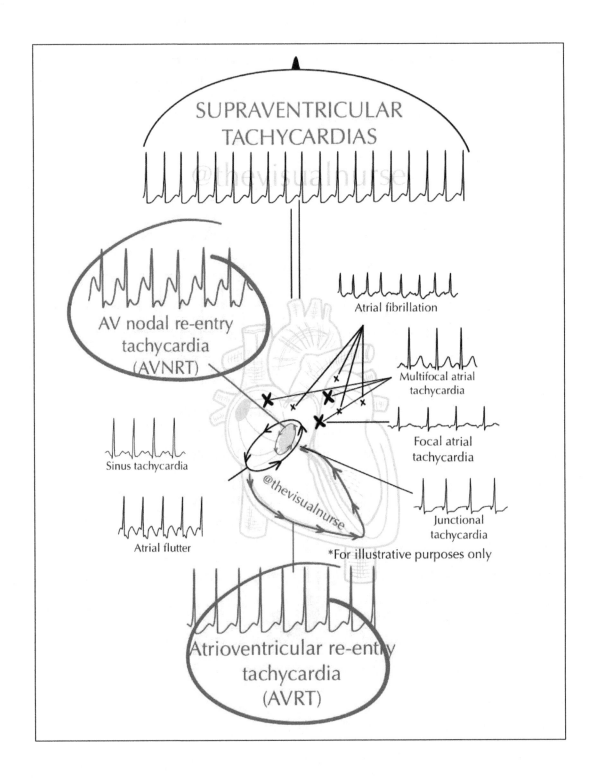

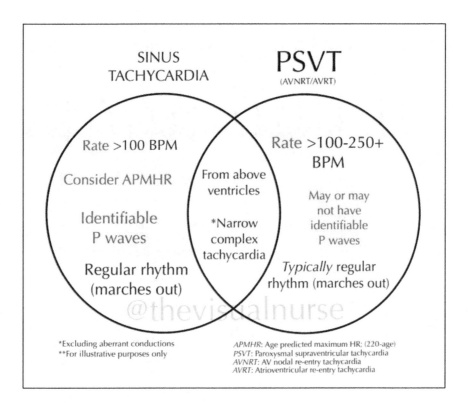

Differentiating sinus tachycardia from SVT is a difficult task for beginners. If you cannot tell where the T waves ends and the P wave begins, you may want to lead more toward SVT (consider situation and age predicted max HR). Regularity of the rhythm plays a big role in differentiating rapid A-fib from AVNRT/AVRT (below).

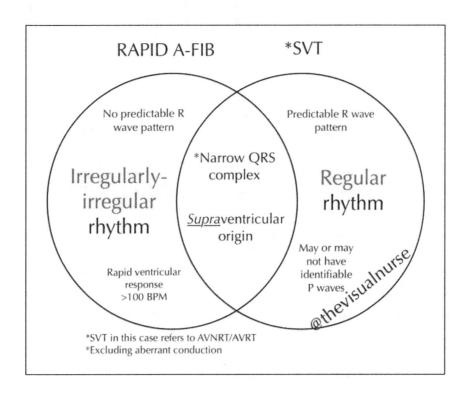

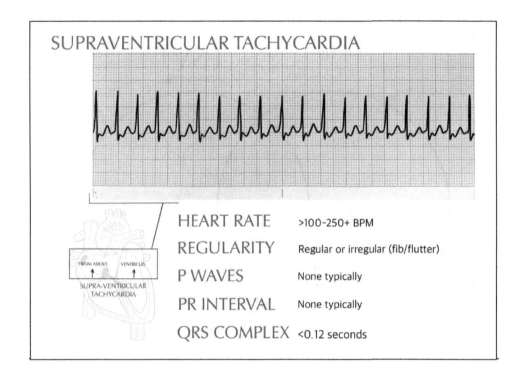

SUPRAVENTRICULAR TACHYCARDIA

HEART RATE	>100-250+ BPM
REGULARITY	Regular or irregular (fib/flutter)
P WAVES	None typically
PR INTERVAL	None typically
QRS COMPLEX	<0.12 seconds

SUPRAVENTRICULAR TACHYCARDIA

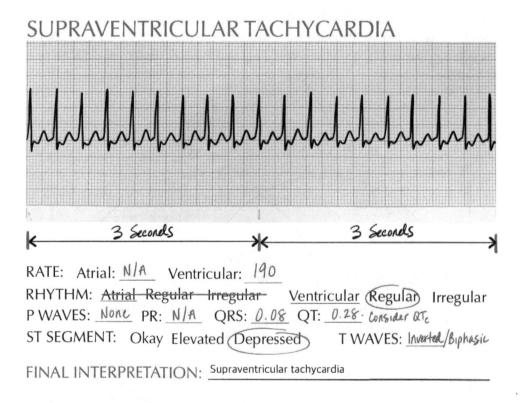

3 Seconds   3 Seconds

RATE: Atrial: N/A   Ventricular: 190

RHYTHM: ~~Atrial Regular Irregular~~   Ventricular (Regular) Irregular

P WAVES: None PR: N/A QRS: 0.08 QT: 0.28 Consider QTc

ST SEGMENT: Okay Elevated (Depressed)   T WAVES: Inverted/Biphasic

FINAL INTERPRETATION: Supraventricular tachycardia

Follow along with the sample rhythm interpretation above using the concepts that we've discussed to this point.

ECG RATES

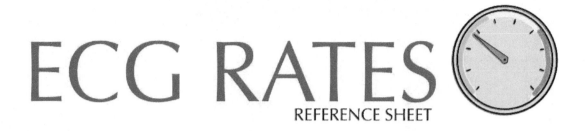

REFERENCE SHEET

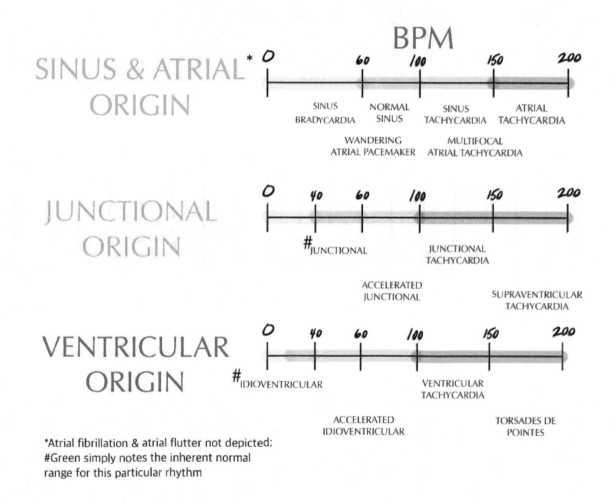

*Atrial fibrillation & atrial flutter not depicted;
#Green simply notes the inherent normal
range for this particular rhythm

This concludes the junctional origin arrhythmias. Next up we'll take a look at rhythms and arrhythmias of ventricular origin as we progress from top to bottom in our examination of potential cardiac conduction sites.

JUNCTIONAL ORIGIN PRACTICE

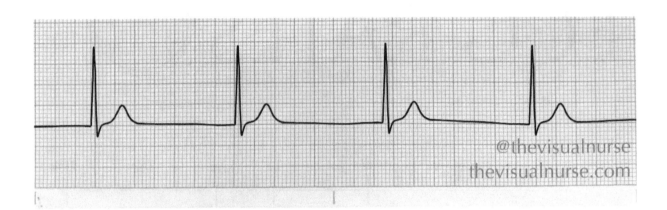

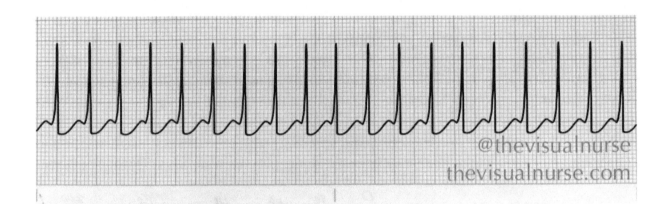

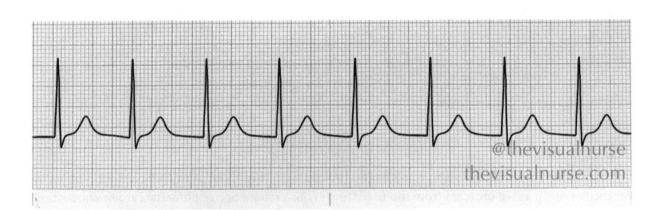

Turn to the "Rhythm strips answer key" section in the back of the book to check your answers!

CHAPTER 8: ARRHYTHMIAS OF VENTRICULAR ORIGIN

IDIOVENTRICULAR

ACCELERATED
IDIOVENTRICULAR

VENTRICULAR
TACHYCARDIA

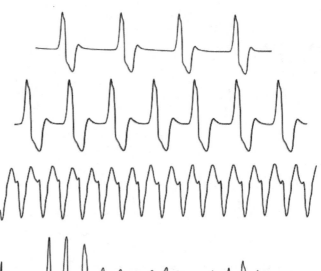

TORSADES

VENTRICULAR
FIBRILLATION

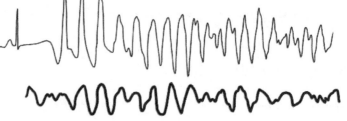

ASYSTOLE

Ventricular origin and ventricular ecopty overview

VENTRICULAR ORIGIN

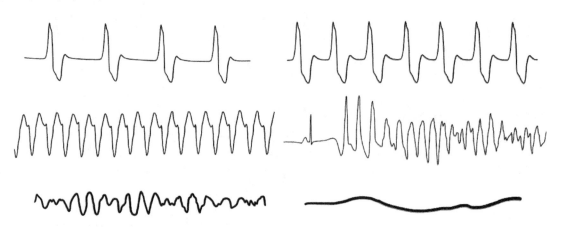

What is ventricular origin?

The ventricles: the final frontier.

What does this mean?

The intrinsic rate for the ventricles as an inherent *pacemaker* is about 20 – 40 beats per minute but this may vary[17,22,24]. Why does this matter? Well, you've probably heard this somewhere before but the reason we largely care about most arrhythmias is the end effect on total cardiac output.

Why should we care?

Rapid identification of ventricular arrhythmias is paramount. The key characteristics to look for are a lack of P waves that are initiating the arrhythmia, and a wide QRS. Hmm. Why would the QRS be wide? We'll talk about that too. Some of these arrhythmias are regular (remember your R-R interval) and some are not. We'll look at this soon but first; we need to understand ventricular *ectopy* and its relation to ventricular *arrhythmias*. Let's start with the single premature ventricular contraction (PVC).

Premature ventricular contractions

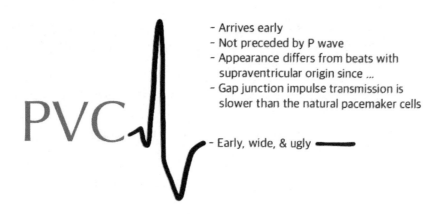

- Arrives early
- Not preceded by P wave
- Appearance differs from beats with supraventricular origin since ...
- Gap junction impulse transmission is slower than the natural pacemaker cells

- Early, wide, & ugly

What is a premature ventricular contraction?

First, we'll look at premature ventricular contractions. A single PVC stems from a singular irritable focus (site) in the ventricles. As the name suggests, they come early and from the ventricle (either left or right).

What does this mean?

When these occur, a single premature ectopic complex that is EARLY, WIDE (>0.12s), and UGLY presents on the ECG strip. These ventricular complexes appear different from the underlying rhythm's QRS complex because they are not following the same rules of downstream stimulation. Think of the normal cardiac conduction tract from the SA node down to the purkinje fibers as a fast track to the ventricles in which these highly conductive and specialized cells quickly send the signal where it needs to go. Instead of the impulse arriving at the ventricles from the SA to AV node, to bundle of His, etcetera... these depolarization waveforms are initiated elsewhere in the ventricle, which includes the Purkinje system and/or the ventricular myocardium[18].

Why should we care?

This means the impulse now must travel through the cardiac contractile and conductive tissue to activate the entire lower chambers. Additionally, this impulse also travels from one ventricle to the other, instead of simultaneous activation through the His system above, contributing to a longer depolarization time[18]. This is possible through the use of gap junctions, but muscle tissue is thick and it doesn't conduct as efficiently as the fast-track cells. The result is a wide abnormal QRS complex (greater than 0.12 seconds in duration) instead of a thin, tight QRS complex (less than 0.12 seconds in duration). Expect the associated T wave to present in the opposite direction of the QRS.

Stimulation or irritation of the myocardium may elicit PVCs. Causes may include coronary perfusion defects, stimulants use, electrolyte imbalances, and reduced ejection fractions/heart failure[18]. PVCs are typically treated if they're increasing in frequency and/or producing symptoms which may range from palpitations to lightheadedness. Now that we understand what PVCs are, we'll describe them based upon appearance in the sections that follow.

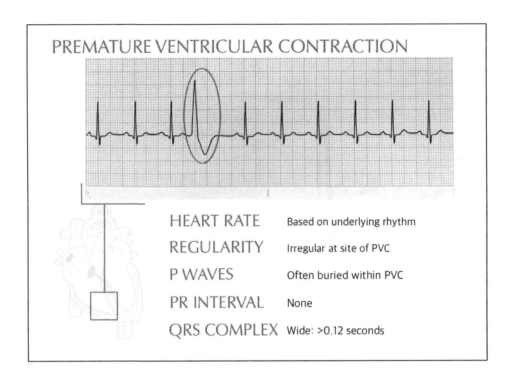

PREMATURE VENTRICULAR CONTRACTION

HEART RATE	Based on underlying rhythm
REGULARITY	Irregular at site of PVC
P WAVES	Often buried within PVC
PR INTERVAL	None
QRS COMPLEX	Wide: >0.12 seconds

PREMATURE VENTRICULAR CONTRACTION

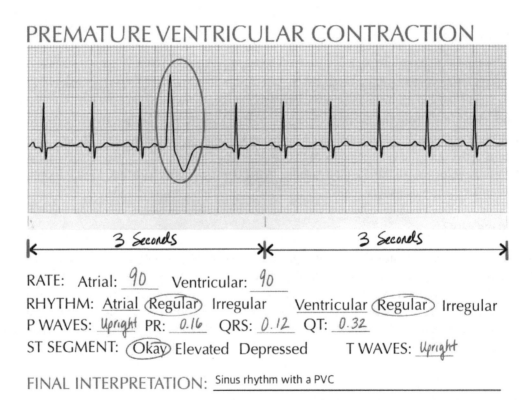

3 Seconds   3 Seconds

RATE: Atrial: _90_   Ventricular: _90_

RHYTHM: Atrial (Regular) Irregular   Ventricular (Regular) Irregular

P WAVES: _Upright_ PR: _0.16_   QRS: _0.12_   QT: _0.32_

ST SEGMENT: (Okay) Elevated Depressed   T WAVES: _Upright_

FINAL INTERPRETATION: _Sinus rhythm with a PVC_

Note that when describing the atrial and ventricular rate we're doing so for the underlying rhythm, ignoring the PVC. Additionally, for rate calculation we're using the 6 second strip method. Advanced readers may notice however that the actual heart rate would fall around 90-100 BPM by the big box method and approximately 100 BPM by the small box method (Chapter 4).

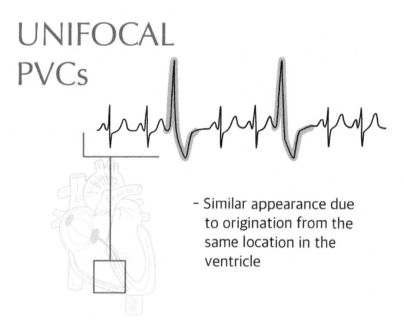

UNIFOCAL PVCs

- Similar appearance due to origination from the same location in the ventricle

What are they?

The same general criteria previously described for PVCs is true for unifocal PVCs.

What does this mean?

Unifocal (Uni: *singular*; focal: focus, or *site*) is a description indicating that PVCs present are assumed to be generated by the same focus, or area in the ventricles.

Why should we care?

Similar waveform appearances tell us the electrode sensing the impulse is receiving the same view. This produces similar ECG waveforms and happens because the impulses are assumed to originate from the same site. By comparison, multifocal or multiform PVCs which are presented next, arise from differing sites within the ventricles. To properly describe ectopy of any type we have to first understand the concept of differing ectopic origins resulting in differing ectopic appearances.

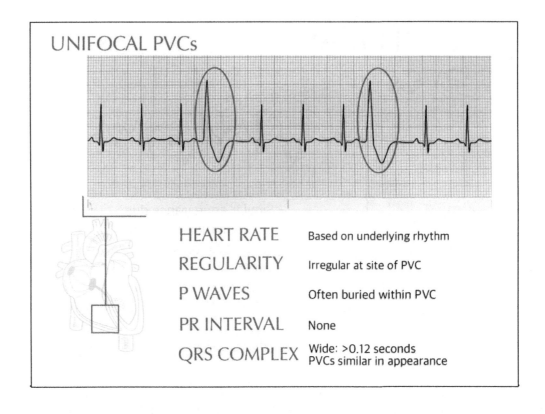

UNIFOCAL PVCs

HEART RATE	Based on underlying rhythm
REGULARITY	Irregular at site of PVC
P WAVES	Often buried within PVC
PR INTERVAL	None
QRS COMPLEX	Wide: >0.12 seconds PVCs similar in appearance

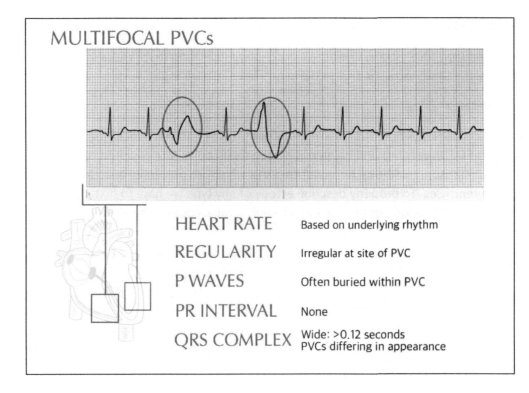

MULTIFOCAL PVCs

HEART RATE	Based on underlying rhythm
REGULARITY	Irregular at site of PVC
P WAVES	Often buried within PVC
PR INTERVAL	None
QRS COMPLEX	Wide: >0.12 seconds PVCs differing in appearance

UNIFOCAL PVCs

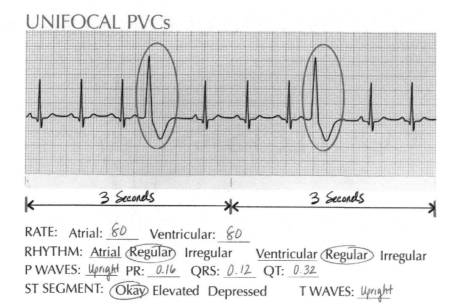

RATE: Atrial: _80_ Ventricular: _80_
RHYTHM: Atrial (Regular) Irregular   Ventricular (Regular) Irregular
P WAVES: _Upright_ PR: _0.16_ QRS: _0.12_ QT: _0.32_
ST SEGMENT: (Okay) Elevated Depressed   T WAVES: _Upright_

FINAL INTERPRETATION: _Sinus rhythm with unifocal PVCs_

Follow along with the sample rhythm interpretation above using the concepts that we've discussed to this point. As before, when describing rhythm regularity we're doing so for the underlying rhythm, ignoring the PVCs.

MULTIFOCAL PVCs

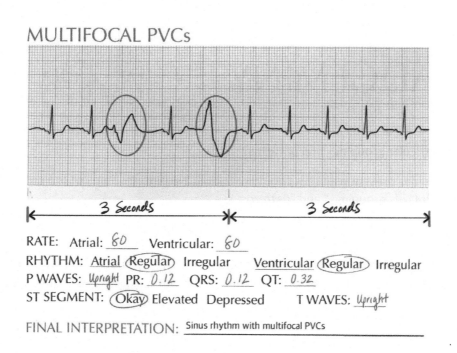

RATE: Atrial: _80_ Ventricular: _80_
RHYTHM: Atrial (Regular) Irregular   Ventricular (Regular) Irregular
P WAVES: _Upright_ PR: _0.12_ QRS: _0.12_ QT: _0.32_
ST SEGMENT: (Okay) Elevated Depressed   T WAVES: _Upright_

FINAL INTERPRETATION: _Sinus rhythm with multifocal PVCs_

Next up, let's look at the various *groupings* and *patterns* associated with ventricular ectopy

VENTRICULAR ECTOPIC GROUPS & PATTERNS

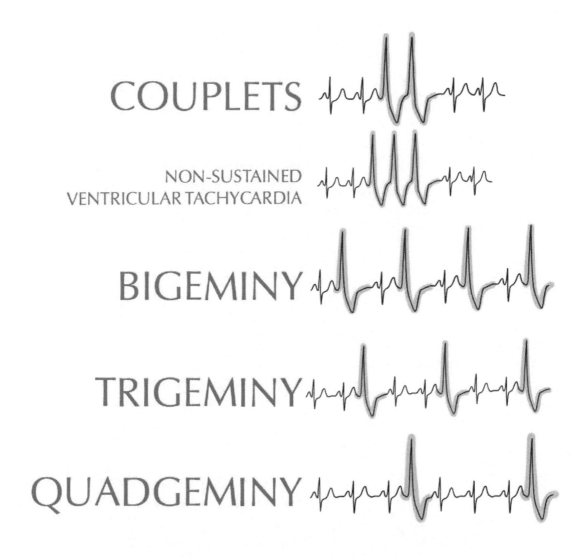

COUPLETS

NON-SUSTAINED
VENTRICULAR TACHYCARDIA

BIGEMINY

TRIGEMINY

QUADGEMINY

What are the ventricular groupings and patterns?

Ventricular ectopy may present with or without an identifiable pattern. Think of premature ventricular contractions in terms of "groupings" and "patterns".

What does this mean?

Groupings of ventricular ectopy include ventricular couplets as well as non-sustained ventricular tachycardia (NSVT). *Patterns* of PVCs by comparison include ventricular bigeminy, trigeminy, and quadgeminy.

Why should we care?

To communicate rhythms and ectopic beats that deviate from "normal" we must have an understanding of the definitions associated with each. The sections that follow will provide these descriptions.

COUPLET
PVCs

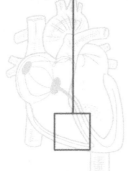

- PVCs that occur as a pair
  of two
- Do not confuse with
  PVCs in bigeminy

What are ventricular couplets?

Ventricular couplets. They come in pairs.

What does this mean?

Think of two people that show up to a party together. The underlying rhythm in the example above is a normal sinus rhythm with a small interruption, the brief interruption being the couplet. The couplet appears when they walk through the door together. After everyone says hello, the party goes on as before (sinus is resumed).

Why should we care?

Be careful not to confuse this with ventricular bigeminy. For now, think couplet = couple. Ventricular ectopy may be idiopathic. It may also be the result of heart disease, excessive caffeine or stimulant use, or any number of issues previously mentioned[18]. Ventricular couplets that are increasing in frequency may also represent ischemic changes or an irritable heart. If this is a change from baseline, assess the patient and report to the provider.

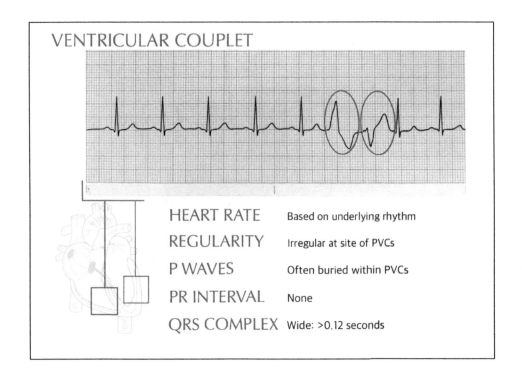

VENTRICULAR COUPLET

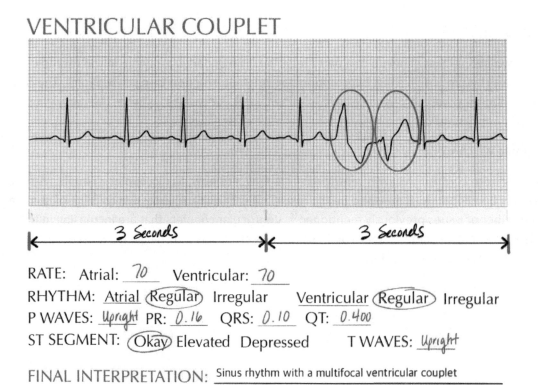

RATE: Atrial: 70   Ventricular: 70
RHYTHM: Atrial (Regular) Irregular   Ventricular (Regular) Irregular
P WAVES: Upright PR: 0.16 QRS: 0.10 QT: 0.400
ST SEGMENT: (Okay) Elevated Depressed   T WAVES: Upright

FINAL INTERPRETATION: Sinus rhythm with a multifocal ventricular couplet

Remember, ventricular couplets may come from the same area of the ventricles which would produce two similar PVC waveforms (unifocal). However, as shown above you may see PVCs with two different appearances (multifocal/multiform).

Non-sustained ventricular tachycardia

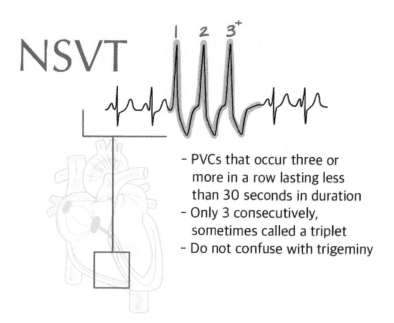

NSVT

- PVCs that occur three or more in a row lasting less than 30 seconds in duration
- Only 3 consecutively, sometimes called a triplet
- Do not confuse with trigeminy

What is non-sustained ventricular tachycardia?

Depending on setting and situation, non-sustained ventricular tachycardia (NSVT) may be benign or may serve as a warning of events to come.

What does this mean?

"Non-sustained" is telling us that the ventricular tachycardia lasts less than 30 seconds before terminating. Ventricular tachycardia tells us that by definition, 3 or more successive PVCs are present. Often you may also hear 3 PVCs in a row referred to as a "triplet" which is fine. Just know that a triplet is 3 PVCs, and 3 or more PVCs consecutively is referred to as ventricular tachycardia by textbook definition[18].

Why should we care?

As you probably guessed, NSVT can be used to describe 4, 5, 6, 7, or even 15+ PVCs in a row if the rhythm terminates prior to 30 seconds. If it lasts greater than 30 seconds, we call this sustained ventricular tachycardia. PVCs may not always appear the same. They may be from the same irritable foci in the ventricles (monomorphic), or they may arise from different foci, appearing different from one another (multifocal, or polymorphic). Non-sustained ventricular tachycardia may be the result of any of the previously mentioned causes associate with PVCs. In any case, NSVT is *not normal* and may represent ischemic changes or an unhappy heart. If this is encountered, assess the patient and report to the provider. We should also expect that lab work will be requested to assess electrolyte values in addition to an updated 12 lead ECG.

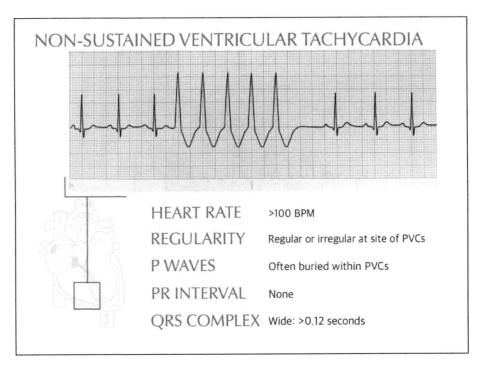

I want to point out that the rhythm cheat sheet above shows unifocal NSVT; the beats are coming from the same site. This makes the NSVT relatively *regular* when marching out the R waves. It is possible to have an *irregular* run of NSVT if the PVCs are multifocal, also known as *polymorphic*.

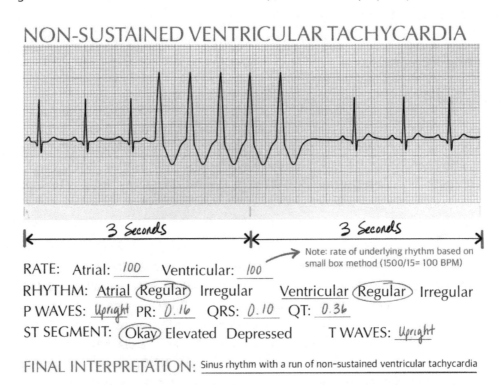

Notice that in the interpretation above, we're describing the rate and regularity of the underlying rhythm, ignoring the ectopy.

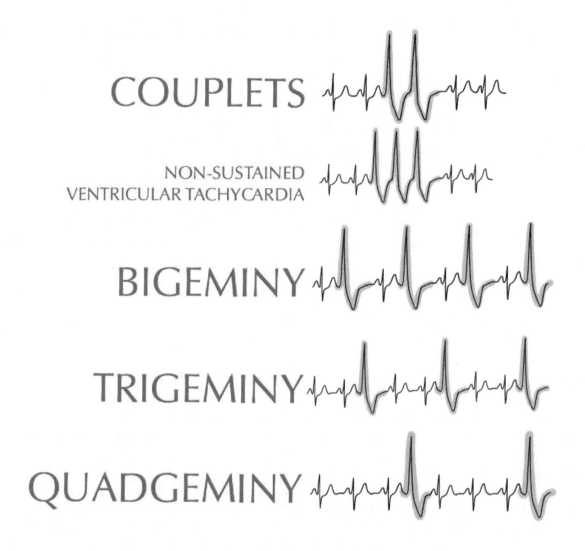

From ventricular groupings, we move to ventricular patterns.

Patterns: Ventricular Bigeminy, Trigeminy, and Quadgeminy describe the pattern in which PVCs are appearing. When first learning these patterns, it's common to confuse couplets with bigeminy and triplets with trigeminy but remember to group them separately. Is it a grouping or a pattern?

Ventricular bigeminy and trigeminy

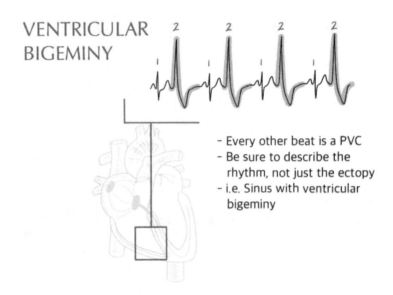

VENTRICULAR BIGEMINY

- Every other beat is a PVC
- Be sure to describe the rhythm, not just the ectopy
- i.e. Sinus with ventricular bigeminy

What is ventricular bigeminy?

The pattern above shows ventricular bigeminy meaning every second beat is a PVC. In ventricular trigeminy every third beat is a PVC. In ventricular quadgeminy every fourth beat is a PVC. Easy, right?

What does this mean?

What's also important is how we address the underlying rhythm. The PVCs are an interruption in the underlying rhythm. Because of this, we should describe the underlying rhythm first (i.e. sinus rhythm) followed by the PVC grouping or pattern present (sinus rhythm with PVCs in bigeminy; or sinus rhythm with a PVC/ventricular couplet).

Why should we care?

As with any ventricular ectopy, this may be the result of previously mentioned causes. Ventricular ectopy that is increasing in frequency may represent ischemic changes or an unhappy heart and if this is a change from baseline, assess the patient and report to the provider. In the pages that follow we'll look at the rhythm cheat sheets and sample rhythm interpretations for these ventricular patterns together.

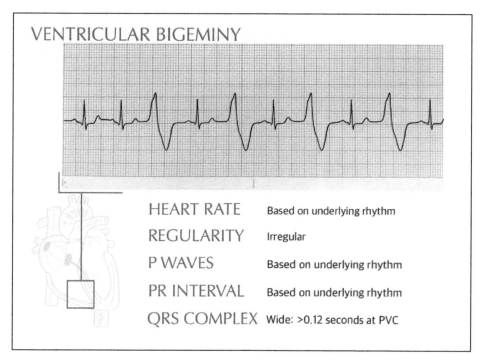

Note that in the cheat sheet above, the arrhythmia is irregular because of the early arrival of each PVC.

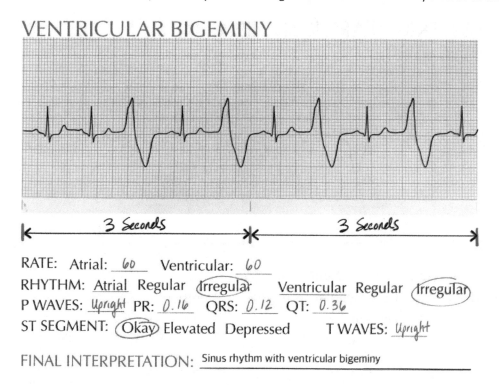

Notice that the baseline interpretation describes the underlying rhythm, followed by the arrhythmia, ventricular bigeminy in this case. Advanced readers will notice that the actual heart rate leading into the ventricular ectopy is around 100 BPM by the small box method (1500 / 15 = 100) however, by the 6 second strip method the sinus heart rate is about 60 BPM for this given strip (6 x 10 = 60 BPM) for the underlying rhythm.

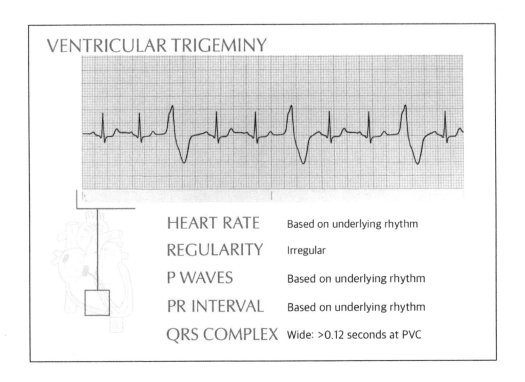

VENTRICULAR TRIGEMINY

HEART RATE	Based on underlying rhythm
REGULARITY	Irregular
P WAVES	Based on underlying rhythm
PR INTERVAL	Based on underlying rhythm
QRS COMPLEX	Wide: >0.12 seconds at PVC

VENTRICULAR TRIGEMINY

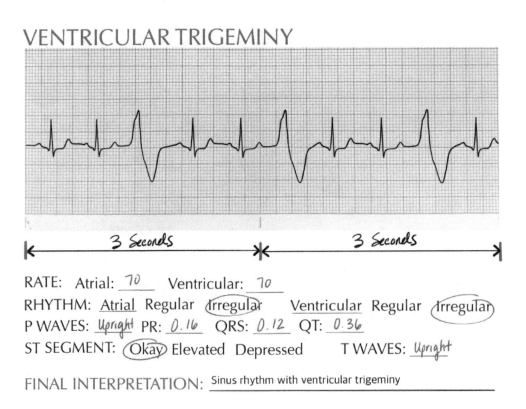

3 Seconds   3 Seconds

RATE: Atrial: _70_   Ventricular: _70_

RHYTHM: Atrial Regular (Irregular)   Ventricular Regular (Irregular)

P WAVES: _Upright_ PR: _0.16_   QRS: _0.12_   QT: _0.36_

ST SEGMENT: (Okay) Elevated Depressed   T WAVES: _Upright_

FINAL INTERPRETATION: _Sinus rhythm with ventricular trigeminy_

Notice that the baseline interpretation describes the underlying rhythm, followed by the arrhythmia, ventricular trigeminy in this case. Advanced readers will notice that the actual heart rate leading into the ventricular ectopy is around 100 BPM by the small box method (1500 / 15 = 100) however, by the 6 second strip method the sinus heart rate is about 70 BPM for this given strip (7 x 10 = 70 BPM).

Arrhythmias of ventricular origin

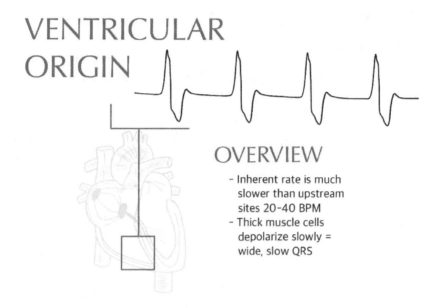

VENTRICULAR ORIGIN

OVERVIEW

- Inherent rate is much slower than upstream sites 20-40 BPM
- Thick muscle cells depolarize slowly = wide, slow QRS

What are ventricular arrhythmias?

We've covered ventricular ectopy. Now we turn to the ventricular *arrhythmias.* Think of these as a sort of maintained rhythm or arrhythmia originating from the ventricles.

What does this mean?

The single site ventricular rhythms include idioventricular (IV), accelerated idioventricular (AIVR), and monomorphic ventricular tachycardia (VT). There is no identifiable P wave in most cases (although the atria will be depolarized retrograde), the QRS will appear wide and bizarre, and the R-to-R interval will relatively march out as a regular rhythm. By comparison, *polymorphic* ventricular tachycardia, torsades de pointes, and ventricular fibrillation are examples of ventricular arrhythmias that arise from more than one site in the ventricles.

Why should we care?

We've mentioned that the intrinsic rate for the ventricles as an inherent *pacemaker* is roughly 20 – 40 beats per minute, but this may vary. Why does this matter? Say it with me, "It all has to do with cardiac output." Let's read on to examine each more closely.

TAKE HOME POINTS:

- ✓ Ventricular rhythms may come from single site or multiple sites
- ✓ The intrinsic rate for the ventricles as an inherent *pacemaker* is 20 – 40 beats per minute but this may vary
- ✓ As with all rhythms and arrhythmias the end effect on total cardiac output is our primary concern

Idioventricular and accelerated idioventricular rhythms

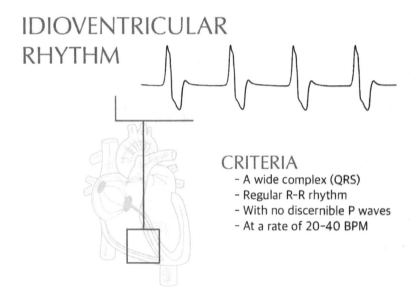

IDIOVENTRICULAR RHYTHM

CRITERIA
- A wide complex (QRS)
- Regular R-R rhythm
- With no discernible P waves
- At a rate of 20-40 BPM

What is an idioventricular rhythm?

Idioventricular and accelerated idioventricular rhythms share the same characteristics above. For these reasons, we'll review them together here.

What does this mean?

These two rhythms present with a wide QRS and no visible P waves, information that tells us the pacemaker site is ventricular in origin. The major problem as you might guess, is associated with the natural inherent rate of the ventricles *as a pacemaker* for the heart. Twenty to forty contractions each minute may not be enough blood flow to perfuse the vital organs, most importantly the brain and heart.

Why should we care?

The major difference for these two ventricular rhythms is maintained in their respective rates. Commonly occurring following the reopening of an occluded coronary artery, these rhythms may be transient in nature and resolve spontaneously[18,22,24]. They may also result from ischemia, or drug therapies. In any case, patient presentation should guide therapy in accordance with hemodynamic stability or instability. Look at the strips that follow to compare the two.

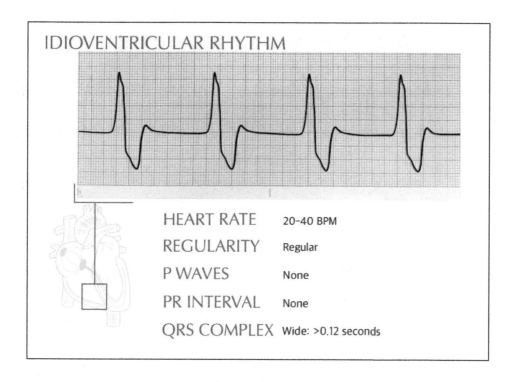

IDIOVENTRICULAR RHYTHM

HEART RATE	20-40 BPM
REGULARITY	Regular
P WAVES	None
PR INTERVAL	None
QRS COMPLEX	Wide: >0.12 seconds

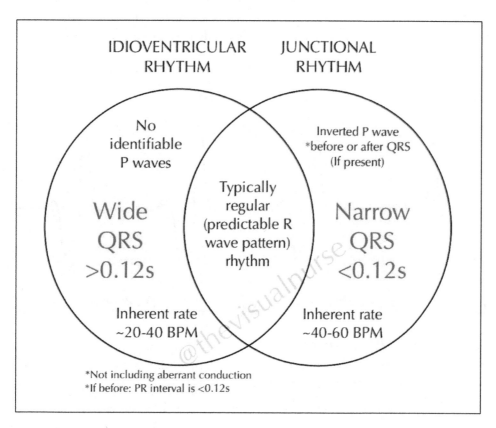

IDIOVENTRICULAR RHYTHM   JUNCTIONAL RHYTHM

No identifiable P waves

Wide QRS >0.12s

Inherent rate ~20-40 BPM

Typically regular (predictable R wave pattern) rhythm

Inverted P wave *before or after QRS (If present)

Narrow QRS <0.12s

Inherent rate ~40-60 BPM

*Not including aberrant conduction
*If before: PR interval is <0.12s

Differentiating idioventricular rhythms from junctional can be tricky for beginners. As the graphic above shows, it's primarily in the width of the QRS.

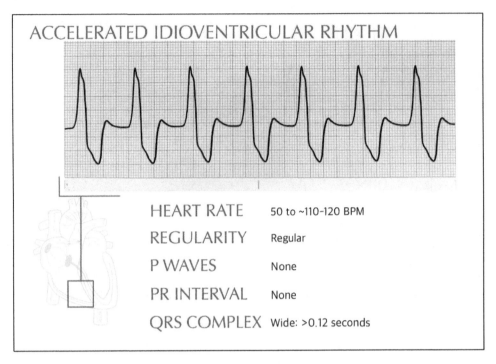

You'll notice that some overlap exists between AIVR and ventricular tachycardia (VT) when we cover VT in the next section. Accelerated idioventricular rhythms are broadly defined as a ventricular *rhythm* exceeding the inherent ventricular rate at a range typically 40 – 60 BPM[24]. Again, this may occur transiently with vessel reperfusion following a heart attack.

IDIOVENTRICULAR RHYTHM

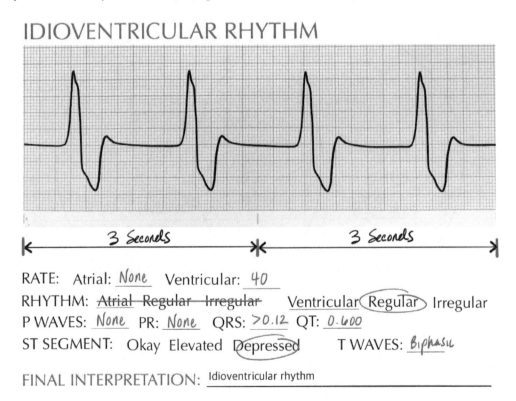

Ventricular tachycardia

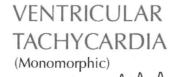

VENTRICULAR
TACHYCARDIA
(Monomorphic)

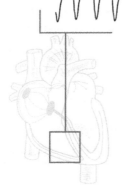

CRITERIA
- A wide complex (QRS) tachycardia with a
- Regular R-R rhythm/interval
- With no discernible P waves
- At a rate greater than 100 BPM

What is ventricular tachycardia?

Ventricular tachycardia is a potentially lethal arrhythmia that may originate from ventricular pacemaker or myocardial cells if condition permits[30].

What does this mean?

The arrhythmia may be *monomorphic*, coming from the same site/foci in the ventricles, or *polymorphic*, arising from different ventricular sites. In line with the principles we've discussed, single site arrhythmias will produce similar looking waveforms, as above. Polymorphic VT demonstrates a wide complex but with alternating appearances. For each there will be no identifiable P waves, and the QRS will appear wide. Rates may in fact range from slightly less than 100 BPM depending upon the mechanism to upwards of 270 BPM[18]. For our purposes and from a bedside nursing perspective we'll be using >100 BPM as our criteria for consistency.

Extremely rapid heart rates may impair ventricular filling time. The coronary arteries feed the heart during diastole. If filling time decreases so does the blood supply to the heart. Additionally, contractions that originate in the ventricles are inefficient contractions. This is due to the concepts covered earlier explaining in part why electrical impulses take much longer to travel through the myocardium when they're initiated by the ventricular muscle versus the cardiac conduction pathway (remember the fast track!).

For these combined reasons, this arrhythmia has the potential to rapidly deteriorate into ventricular fibrillation and death. With ventricular tachycardia, the cardiac workload is greatly *increased* and its blood supply may be greatly *decreased*.

Why should we care?

Causes of ventricular tachycardia may include coronary perfusion defects, electrolyte imbalances (potassium and magnesium in particular), multiple forms of cardiomyopathy, certain drugs, inflammatory diseases, and more[18]. They may also be idiopathic.

Treatment should depend on hemodynamic stability in accordance with current advanced cardiac life support (ACLS) guidelines. The patient may or may not have a pulse. This is important to determine quickly because the treatment for pulseless ventricular tachycardia differs greatly than for stable VT with a pulse. If we're lucky the patient may have a documented history of ventricular arrhythmia due to known cardiomyopathy or other cause, in which case an implantable cardioverter defibrillator (ICD) may already be present. In these cases, the device is programmed to internally "shock" or defibrillate the patient out of the lethal rhythm. Even if this is the case, report this to the provider since additional treatments may be needed if ICD discharges are increasing in frequency.

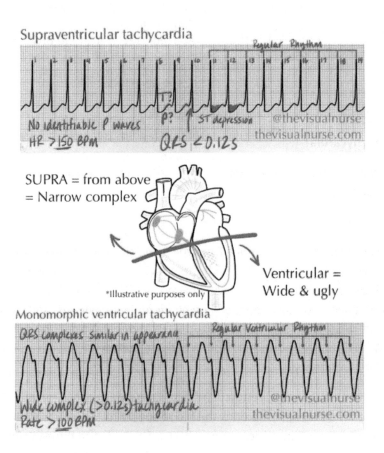

A quick note on VT versus SVT. Look at the width of the QRS. Of course, this does not account for SVT with aberrant conductions which is beyond our scope here. An interesting fact, however, is that regarding prevalence alone, these wide complex tachycardias are in fact ventricular tachycardia around 80% of the time, and this may exceed 90% if the patient has had a previous heart attack prior to tachycardic symptom onset[30].

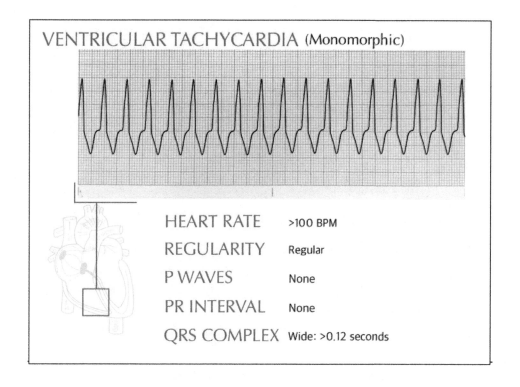

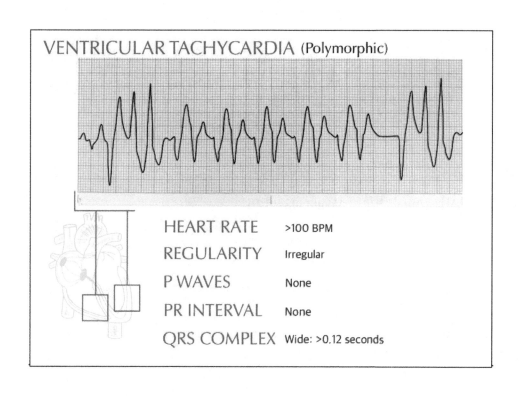

MONOMORPHIC VENTRICULAR TACHYCARDIA

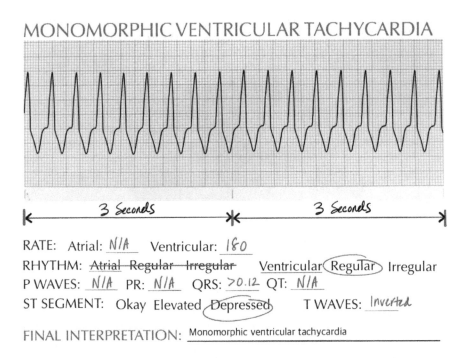

3 Seconds   3 Seconds

RATE: Atrial: _N/A_   Ventricular: _180_
RHYTHM: ~~Atrial Regular Irregular~~   Ventricular (Regular) Irregular
P WAVES: _N/A_ PR: _N/A_ QRS: _>0.12_ QT: _N/A_
ST SEGMENT: Okay Elevated (Depressed)   T WAVES: _Inverted_

FINAL INTERPRETATION: Monomorphic ventricular tachycardia

Follow along with the sample rhythm interpretations above and below using the concepts that we've discussed to this point.

POLYMORPHIC VENTRICULAR TACHYCARDIA

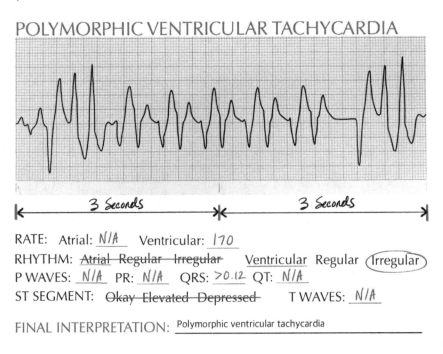

3 Seconds   3 Seconds

RATE: Atrial: _N/A_   Ventricular: _170_
RHYTHM: ~~Atrial Regular Irregular~~   Ventricular Regular (Irregular)
P WAVES: _N/A_ PR: _N/A_ QRS: _>0.12_ QT: _N/A_
ST SEGMENT: ~~Okay Elevated Depressed~~   T WAVES: _N/A_

FINAL INTERPRETATION: Polymorphic ventricular tachycardia

Next up are a few multi-site ventricular arrhythmias: torsades de pointes, and ventricular fibrillation. Asystole will also be presented in the section that follows.

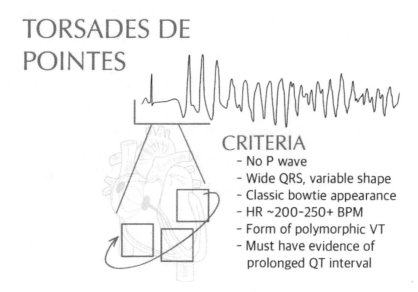

TORSADES DE POINTES

CRITERIA
- No P wave
- Wide QRS, variable shape
- Classic bowtie appearance
- HR ~200-250+ BPM
- Form of polymorphic VT
- Must have evidence of
  prolonged QT interval

What is torsades de pointes?

All torsades de pointes are polymorphic VT but not all polymorphic VT is torsades.

What does this mean?

Torsades de pointes (a twisting of the points; TdP) describes a very specific form of polymorphic VT. The "twisting of the points" to which the name refers describes multiple ventricular ectopic sites rotating around the heart, changing its electrical "axis" as they do so. This occurs at very rapid rates, up to and around 250 beats per minute[17]! Remember, the axis describes the *vector* of the heart which we covered when we learned about positive and negative deflections back in Chapter 2.

If the area of the ventricles initiating the depolarization is constantly rotating and shifting, then you would expect the morphology of the QRS to change along with this! As the electrical foci rotate and spiral around the heart a beautiful but dangerous "bowtie appearance" ventricular tachycardia presents on the rhythm strip.

Why should we care?

Hallmark causes of TdP are low magnesium/potassium levels and a prolonged QT interval[31], although profound bradycardias, heart attack or coronary perfusion defects may precipitate this.

Remember that the QT interval represents complete ventricular depolarization and repolarization. If the QT interval is prolonged, then the T wave extends further from the QRS complex. The heart is electrically sensitive and *refractory* to depolarizing during this phase (T wave) and if a premature ventricular contraction occurs, its R wave just might land on the T wave. When this happens, the heart is sent into this electrically chaotic rhythm resulting from this "R on T" phenomenon.

Causes of long QT syndrome may also include genetic predisposition or electrolyte imbalances[18]. Interestingly, some antiarrhythmic medications that function to prolong this cycle may predispose patients to this. For this reason, medication loading protocols exist in which serial ECGs are taken to monitor the QT interval. As with other forms of VT, patient presentation will guide therapy and determine if medications or electrical therapies (defibrillation) will be used.

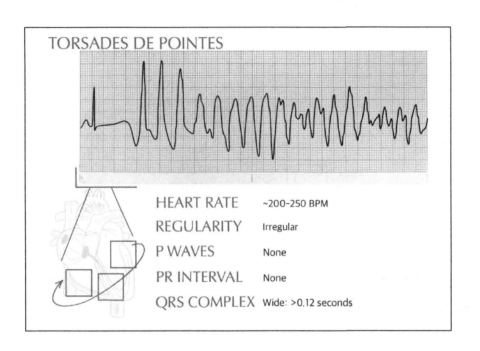

TORSADES DE POINTES

HEART RATE	~200-250 BPM
REGULARITY	Irregular
P WAVES	None
PR INTERVAL	None
QRS COMPLEX	Wide: >0.12 seconds

TORSADES DE POINTES

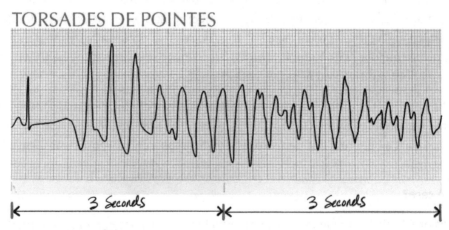

3 Seconds | 3 Seconds

RATE: Atrial: _N/A_ Ventricular: _~200-250_
RHYTHM: ~~Atrial Regular Irregular~~ Ventricular Regular (Irregular)
P WAVES: _N/A_ PR: _N/A_ QRS: _>0.12_ QT: _N/A_
ST SEGMENT: ~~Okay Elevated Depressed~~ T WAVES: _N/A_

FINAL INTERPRETATION: _Polymorphic ventricular tachycardia; Torsades de Pointes_

Ventricular fibrillation

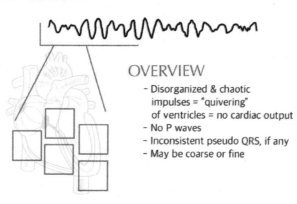

VENTRICULAR
FIBRILLATION

OVERVIEW
- Disorganized & chaotic
  impulses = "quivering"
  of ventricles = no cardiac output
- No P waves
- Inconsistent pseudo QRS, if any
- May be coarse or fine

What is ventricular fibrillation?

Fibrillation = quivering. Recall from our section on atrial fibrillation that this occurrence in the atria may equate to roughly 10-30% loss of total cardiac output. What happens if this is the case in the almighty ventricles?

What does this mean?

The patient will be dead or suffer severe brain injury if not corrected within 3-5 minutes[18]. Like the disorganized activity associated with atrial fibrillation, the ventricles are now fibrillating in a manner that's previously been described as having the appearance of a bag of worms contracting. I know, gross. But I promise that now you'll never forget why with this rhythm, cardiac output is next to zero. If you fail to initiate immediate CPR and advanced cardiac life support protocols, your patient stands zero chance of survival (similar to what their cardiac output is.)

Why should we care?

Causes of ventricular fibrillation include[18]:

- ✓ Cardiac perfusion defects and heart attack
- ✓ Electrolyte disturbances
- ✓ Resultant of deterioration of other lethal arrhythmias
- ✓ Many others

If you encounter this rhythm, your first action is to immediately start CPR and call for help. Defibrillation should be attempted as soon as possible, typically followed by alternating rounds of epinephrine and amiodarone or lidocaine[32] (defer to clinical judgement and facility protocols). Remember, the only way out of V-fib is to D-fib(rillate). Early shocking leads to better outcomes.

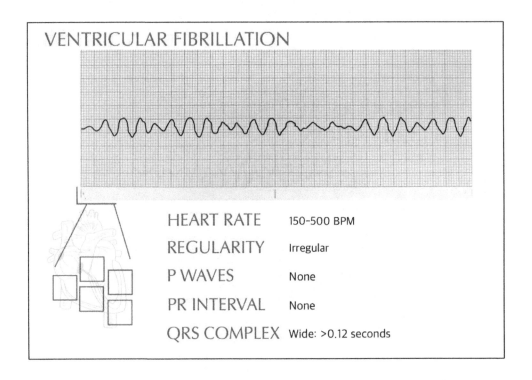

VENTRICULAR FIBRILLATION

HEART RATE	150-500 BPM
REGULARITY	Irregular
P WAVES	None
PR INTERVAL	None
QRS COMPLEX	Wide: >0.12 seconds

VENTRICULAR FIBRILLATION

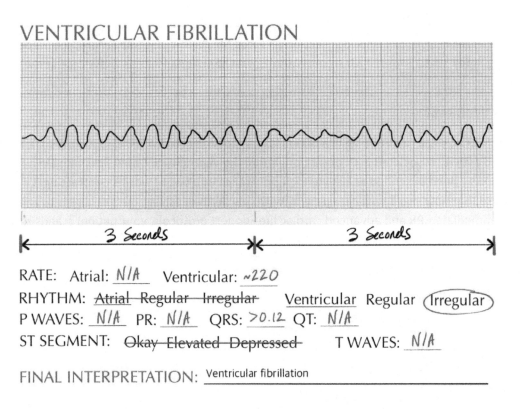

3 Seconds | 3 Seconds

RATE: Atrial: _N/A_   Ventricular: _~220_

RHYTHM: Atrial ~~Regular~~ ~~Irregular~~   Ventricular Regular (Irregular)

P WAVES: _N/A_ PR: _N/A_ QRS: _>0.12_ QT: _N/A_

ST SEGMENT: ~~Okay Elevated Depressed~~   T WAVES: _N/A_

FINAL INTERPRETATION: _Ventricular fibrillation_

Follow along with the sample rhythm interpretation above using the concepts that we've discussed to this point.

ASYSTOLE

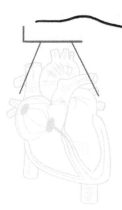

OVERVIEW

- Absence of electrical and
  mechanical (systole) activity
- Absence of cardiac output
- The famed "flat-line"

What is asystole?

The absence of electrical activity in the heart. Asystole refers to the lack of depolarization and contraction (*systole*).

What does this mean?

This is what the medical television shows refer to as "flat-lining" and represents the absence of electrical and mechanical activity in the heart. Asystole is often the result of lethal ventricular rhythm deterioration, including pulseless ventricular tachycardia and ventricular fibrillation. This should be confirmed in more than one lead; an electrode that has fallen off the patient may sometimes mimic this.

Why should we care?

Asystole is the terminal rhythm in cardiac arrest. If encountered, immediate CPR should be performed while initiating the ACLS protocol[32] to include identification of reversible causes referred to as the "H's and T's":

- ✓ Hypovolemia   Tension pneumothorax
- ✓ Hypoxia   Tamponade (cardiac)
- ✓ H+ ion (acidosis)   Toxins
- ✓ Hypo/hyperkalemia   Thrombosis (pulmonary or coronary)
- ✓ Hypothermia

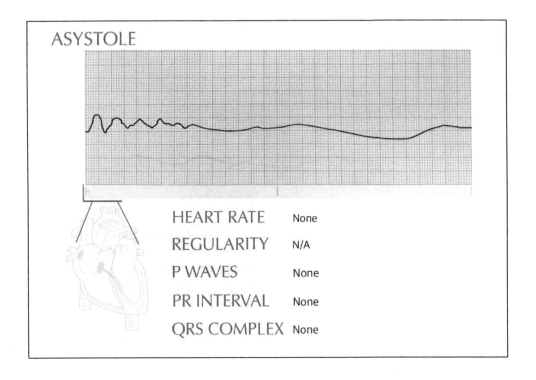

ASYSTOLE

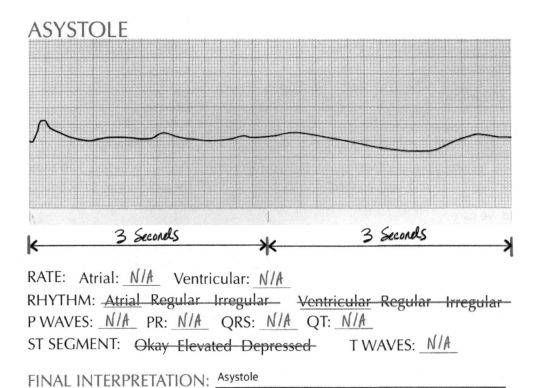

RATE: Atrial: _N/A_ Ventricular: _N/A_

RHYTHM: ~~Atrial Regular Irregular~~ ~~Ventricular Regular Irregular~~

P WAVES: _N/A_ PR: _N/A_ QRS: _N/A_ QT: _N/A_

ST SEGMENT: ~~Okay Elevated Depressed~~ T WAVES: _N/A_

FINAL INTERPRETATION: _Asystole_

Follow along with the sample rhythm interpretation above using the concepts that we've discussed to this point.

ECG RATES
REFERENCE SHEET

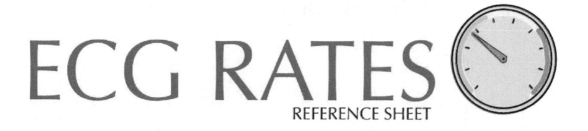

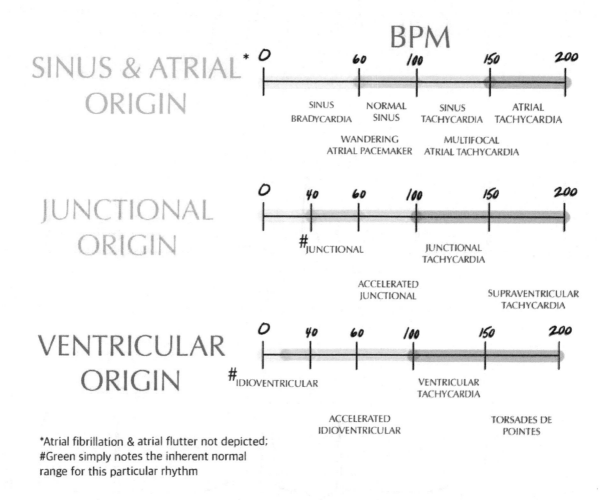

*Atrial fibrillation & atrial flutter not depicted;
#Green simply notes the inherent normal
range for this particular rhythm

This concludes the ventricular origin rhythms and arrhythmias. Next up we'll take a look at the atrioventricular conduction delays and blocks.

VENTRICULAR ORIGIN PRACTICE

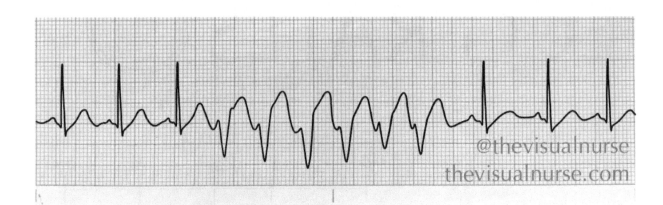

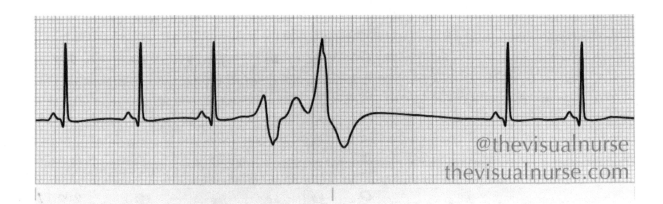

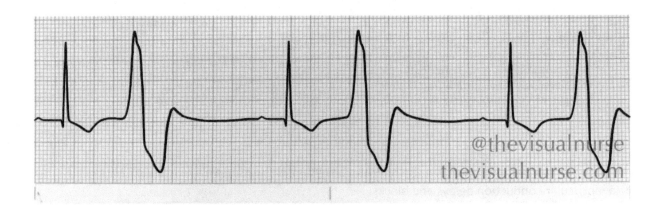

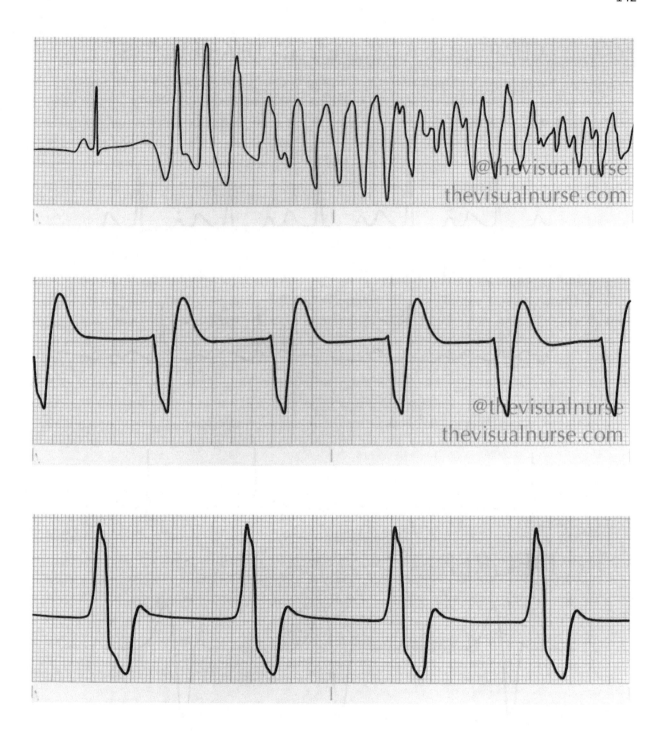

Turn to the "Rhythm strips answer key" section in the back of the book to check your answers!

CHAPTER 9: ATRIOVENTRICULAR BLOCKS

1st DEGREE

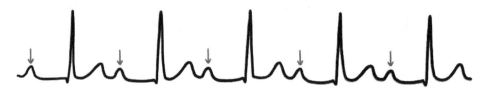

2nd DEGREE (1)

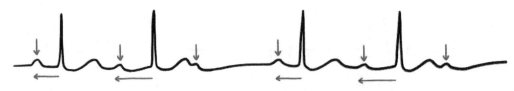

2nd DEGREE (2)

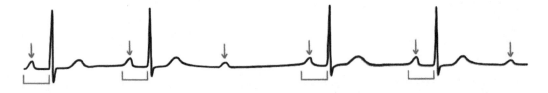

3rd DEGREE

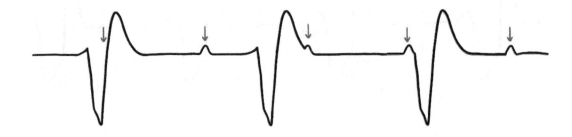

Overview of Atrioventricular blocks

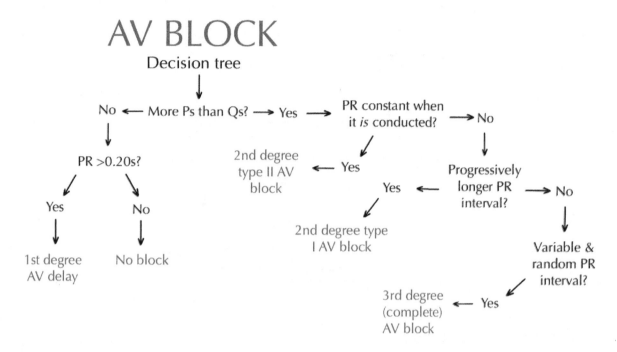

What are heart blocks?

Atrioventricular blocks, commonly referred to as "heart blocks" indicate a disturbance in impulse conduction between the atria and ventricles[22,25].

What does this mean?

Atrioventricular blocks range from harmless to medical emergencies depending upon the severity or grade of the block. For example, first degree heart blocks are typically benign and require no treatment. Comparatively, a third-degree heart block is an emergency and must be evaluated promptly even in patients that are symptom free.

Why should I care?

Your ability to recognize various degrees of AV blocks may save a life, even before symptoms are present.

TAKE HOME POINTS:

- ✓ AV blocks indicate conduction issues between the atria and ventricles
- ✓ Presentations range from harmless to emergent

First degree AV delay

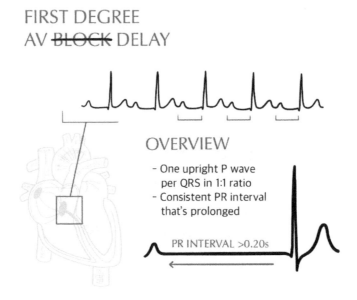

FIRST DEGREE
AV ~~BLOCK~~ DELAY

OVERVIEW

- One upright P wave
  per QRS in 1:1 ratio
- Consistent PR interval
  that's prolonged

PR INTERVAL >0.20s

What is a first-degree AV delay?

The term first degree heart *block* is somewhat misleading.

What does this mean?

A first-degree conduction abnormality involves an *exaggerated* delay of the sinus impulse commonly at the level of the AV node rather than a true block. The word block suggests that impulses are not being conducted but this is not the case with first degree AV blocks. In fact, each impulse is conducted to the ventricles in a 1:1 conduction ratio.

Remember that the normal range for the PR interval is 0.12 to 0.20 seconds. The criteria for first degree AV blocks are that each sinus impulse is transmitted to the ventricles and the PR interval is greater than 0.20 seconds although measures may exceed 0.30 seconds[33]. This conduction delay may occur in either the AV node itself (more common) or in the His-Purkinje system.

Why should we care?

We should consider our patient population when we encounter this conduction delay. First degree AV blocks may be a normal variant in younger and active populations simply due to an enhanced vagal tone at rest. Beta blocking medications are also common culprits. In older patients however, fibrotic changes, heart disease, and other disorders may lead to this abnormality[33]. Regardless of etiology, documentation of this conduction delay is important in order to monitor for changes over time and for potential progression to higher degree AV blocks (i.e. second and third degree). As for recognition, remember *"If your Q's are far from P, then you have a first-degree."*

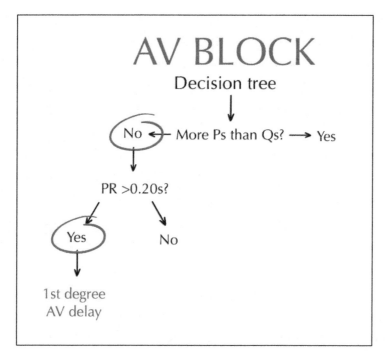

Review the portion of the AV block decision tree above that leads us to the determination of first-degree AV delay.

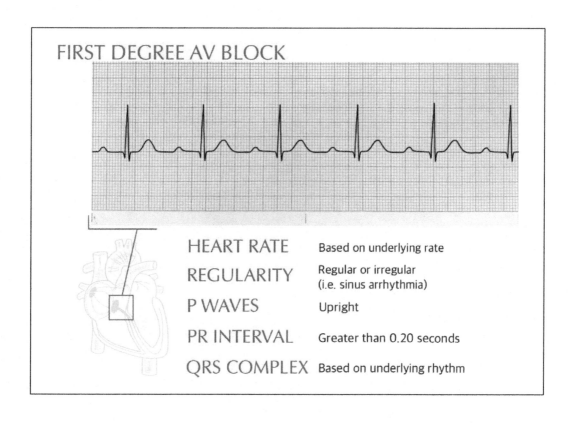

FIRST DEGREE AV BLOCK

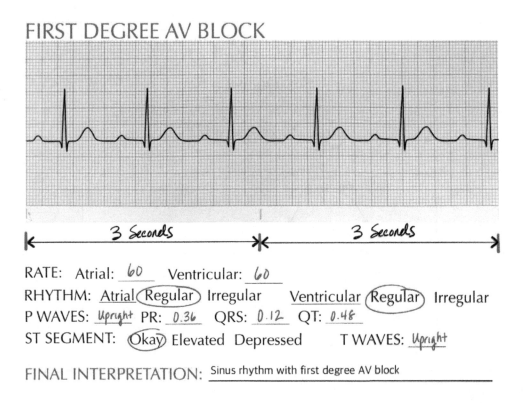

3 Seconds ⟷ 3 Seconds

RATE: Atrial: _60_   Ventricular: _60_

RHYTHM: Atrial (Regular) Irregular   Ventricular (Regular) Irregular

P WAVES: _Upright_ PR: _0.36_   QRS: _0.12_ QT: _0.48_

ST SEGMENT: (Okay) Elevated Depressed   T WAVES: _Upright_

FINAL INTERPRETATION: _Sinus rhythm with first degree AV block_

Follow along with the sample rhythm interpretation above using the concepts that we've discussed to this point.

Second degree Type I AV block

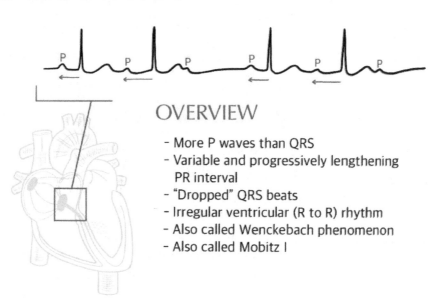

SECOND DEGREE
AV BLOCK TYPE 1

OVERVIEW

- More P waves than QRS
- Variable and progressively lengthening
  PR interval
- "Dropped" QRS beats
- Irregular ventricular (R to R) rhythm
- Also called Wenckebach phenomenon
- Also called Mobitz I

What is a second-degree type I AV block?

Second degree AV blocks can be further categorized as Type I or Type II.

What does this mean?

Following normal sinus impulse generation, electrical conduction must travel through the atria to the AV node. Similar to the first-degree AV block, a second-degree type I block (also called Wenckebach or Mobitz I) may result from an excess in vagal tone or other more serious causes[25]. Additionally, beta blockers, calcium channel blockers, and anti-arrhythmic drugs may lead to this conduction abnormality which is often a harmless and well tolerated variant[24].

In a Mobitz I the relative refractory period (relating to time needed to re-polarize for the next beat) of the AV node is progressively lengthening[24]. This happens until the absolute refractory period is encountered. When this happens a single QRS complex is not conducted or is "dropped" allowing time for the AV node to reset. Often, this is also described as an AV node that's becoming progressively "fatigued" until it finally drops a QRS to reset.

Why should we care?

In order to rapidly differentiate Mobitz I from Mobitz II, first you'll quickly notice that the R to R interval of your narrow QRS is irregular. When you see this you'll attempt to locate your P waves. Once you've located your P waves you should examine the PR interval. Is it progressively getting longer until a QRS is dropped? If yes, then you have a Mobitz I. Remember, *"Longer, longer, longer, drop! Then you have a Wenckebach."*

Take a look at the chart below which we'll review again in the next section on Mobitz II heart blocks.

SECOND DEGREE HEART BLOCKS

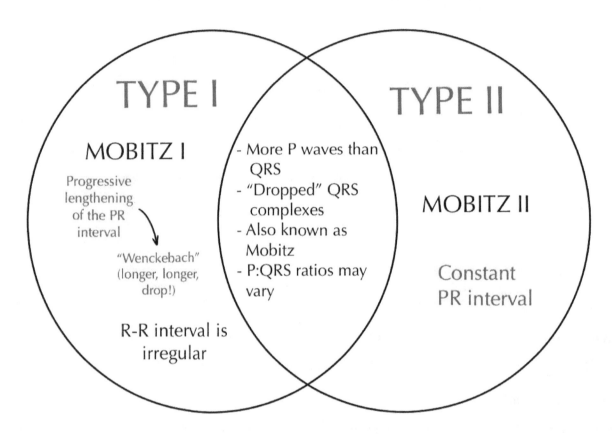

TYPE I

MOBITZ I

Progressive lengthening of the PR interval

"Wenckebach" (longer, longer, drop!)

R-R interval is irregular

- More P waves than QRS
- "Dropped" QRS complexes
- Also known as Mobitz
- P:QRS ratios may vary

TYPE II

MOBITZ II

Constant PR interval

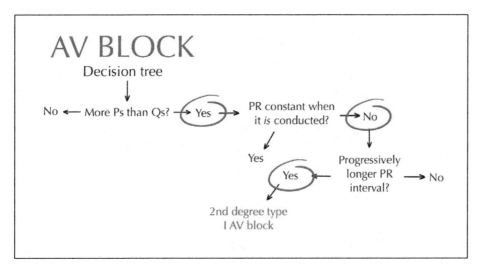

Next, review the portion of the AV block decision tree above that leads us to the determination of second-degree type I AV block.

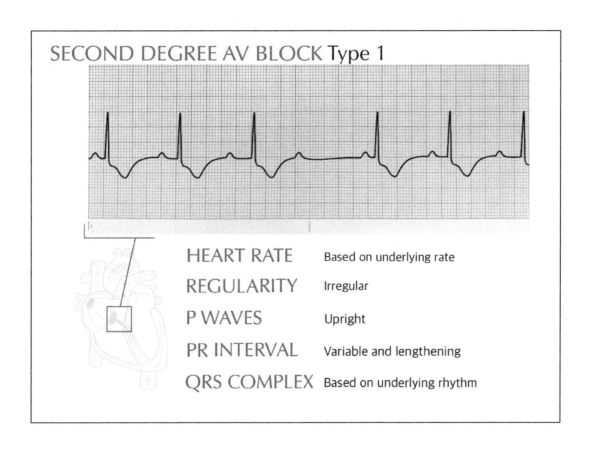

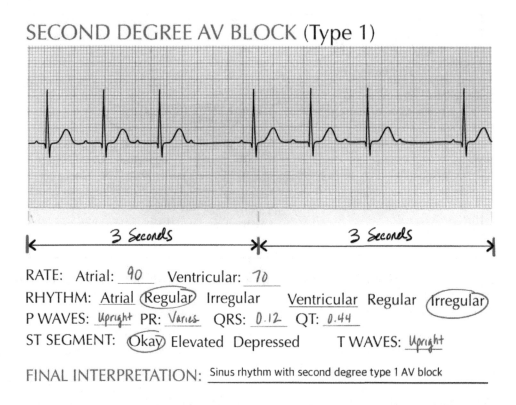

SECOND DEGREE AV BLOCK (Type 1)

3 Seconds — **3 Seconds**

RATE: Atrial: _90_ Ventricular: _70_

RHYTHM: Atrial (Regular) Irregular   Ventricular Regular (Irregular)

P WAVES: Upright PR: Varies QRS: 0.12 QT: 0.44

ST SEGMENT: (Okay) Elevated Depressed   T WAVES: Upright

FINAL INTERPRETATION: _Sinus rhythm with second degree type 1 AV block_

Follow along with the sample rhythm interpretation above using the concepts that we've discussed to this point.

Second degree Type II AV block

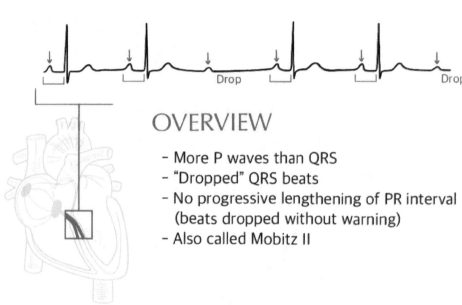

SECOND DEGREE
AV BLOCK TYPE 2

OVERVIEW

- More P waves than QRS
- "Dropped" QRS beats
- No progressive lengthening of PR interval
  (beats dropped without warning)
- Also called Mobitz II

What is a second-degree type II AV block?

Second degree AV blocks can be further categorized as Type I or Type II.

What does this mean?

Following normal sinus impulse generation, the electrical conduction must travel through the atria to the AV node. Whereas second degree type I AV blocks are commonly a result of AV node "fatigability", type II blocks are more commonly associated with issues relating to the His-purkinje system below the AV node[34]. Mobitz II rarely occurs independent of structural heart disease or fibrosis of the heart[24].

On the ECG you'll first notice that the R to R interval may be regular or irregular. Next, you'll quickly attempt to locate P waves. Once you locate the P waves, you'll evaluate the PR interval. If the PR interval is *constant* for each P wave that leads to a ventricular (QRS) contraction, you're looking at a second-degree *type II* AV block. This ECG presentation is a result of the sporadic non-conduction of P waves to the ventricles which occurs without discernible warning. An exception to this would be a 2:1 AV block in which every other P wave results in a ventricular depolarization. In this case, there is insufficient information to tell if the PR interval is prolonging prior to the dropped QRS complex so we simply state presence of 2:1 AV block.

SECOND DEGREE HEART BLOCKS

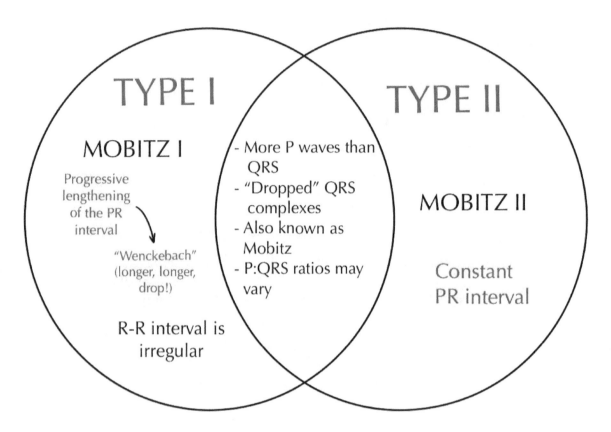

TYPE I

MOBITZ I

Progressive lengthening of the PR interval

"Wenckebach" (longer, longer, drop!)

R-R interval is irregular

- More P waves than QRS
- "Dropped" QRS complexes
- Also known as Mobitz
- P:QRS ratios may vary

TYPE II

MOBITZ II

Constant PR interval

Why should we care?

Patients may be asymptomatic or may present with symptoms ranging from lightheadedness to syncope. If you encounter this rhythm, assess your patient and notify the provider. Mobitz II AV blocks have the potential to progress to complete heart blocks and death if unrecognized and left untreated[22,24].

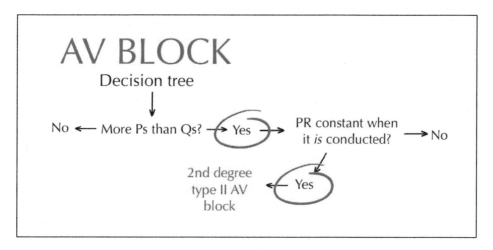

Review the portion of the AV block decision tree above that leads us to the determination of second-degree type II AV block.

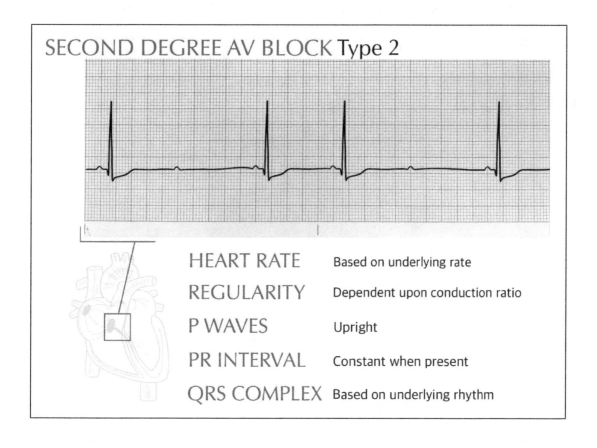

SECOND DEGREE AV BLOCK (Type 2)

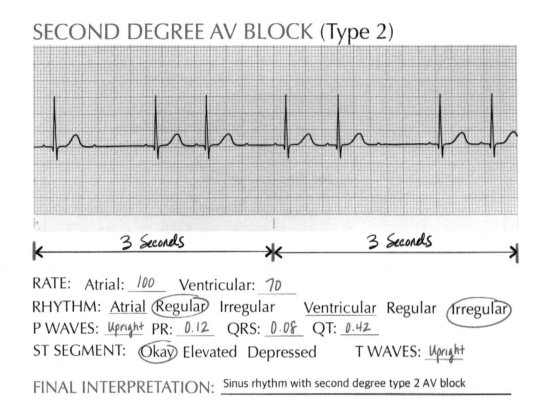

3 Seconds   3 Seconds

RATE: Atrial: _100_   Ventricular: _70_

RHYTHM: Atrial (Regular) Irregular   Ventricular Regular (Irregular)

P WAVES: _Upright_ PR: _0.12_   QRS: _0.08_   QT: _0.42_

ST SEGMENT: (Okay) Elevated Depressed   T WAVES: _Upright_

FINAL INTERPRETATION: _Sinus rhythm with second degree type 2 AV block_

Follow along with the sample rhythm interpretation above using the concepts that we've discussed to this point.

Third degree AV block

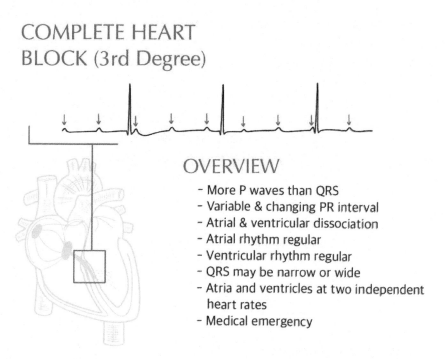

COMPLETE HEART
BLOCK (3rd Degree)

OVERVIEW

- More P waves than QRS
- Variable & changing PR interval
- Atrial & ventricular dissociation
- Atrial rhythm regular
- Ventricular rhythm regular
- QRS may be narrow or wide
- Atria and ventricles at two independent heart rates
- Medical emergency

What is a complete heart block?

A complete heart block is a medical emergency.

What does this mean?

For a typical cardiac cycle, a sinus impulse initiates a wave of depolarization that progresses through the AV node and into the His-purkinje system. This should at a ratio of 1:1 meaning the ventricles contract once for every atrial contraction at a rate of 60 – 100 beats per minute. Why? Because the sinus node depolarizes (normally) at this rate.

Recall that the inherent rate of the ventricles on their own without input from a supraventricular pacemaker is roughly 20 – 40 beats per minute. What do you guess would happen if the connection between the atria and ventricles were lost?

In the case of a complete heart block this is exactly what's occurring. The atria are depolarizing at their normal inherent rate. The ventricles are also depolarizing at their normal inherent rate (exceptions exist, i.e. atrial fibrillation or other atrial arrhythmia with complete AV block). Neither can "see" what the other is doing because the connection has been lost. The consequence is determined by the ventricular rate[24].

It's as if the atria are thinking "Those ventricles sure have got it easy. I send the impulse and all they have to do is respond when they see it. They don't even have to think about it." Meanwhile, the ventricles are thinking "Good thing the heart has us to pick up the slack for that good-for-nothing SA node." Meanwhile, the truth is that both are doing what they think is the right thing, only without any communication whatsoever with the other.

The result is a sinus (or other atrial) rate averaging 60 – 100 beats per minute and a ventricular rate averaging 20 – 40 beats per minute if the ventricles/purkinje system initiates the ventricular activity. The QRS is not always wide necessarily. If the AV junction picks up the escape rhythm before the ventricles, you may still have a narrow QRS at slightly higher rate that is still completely dissociated with the atria.

COMPLETE HEART BLOCK:
the QRS isn't always wide

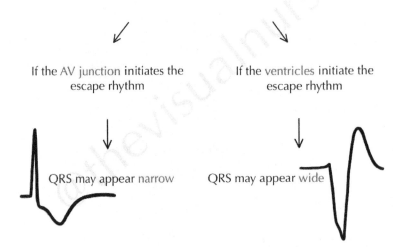

The PR interval will be *variable* and changing with each heartbeat. Any two PR intervals that measure the same are occurring simply by coincidence. Additionally, the P to P intervals should march out relatively regularly as will the ventricular R to R intervals due to the fact that each is capable of providing rhythmic stimuli based on their respective intrinsic rates.

Now, which beats allow for blood perfusion of the entire body including the head and neck; atrial or ventricular? Yes, ventricular! Also, remember why we care about any of the rhythms we've seen to this point... because of their effect on *total cardiac output!* And this is the danger of a ventricular rate between 20 and 40 BPM if initiated below the level of the AV junction. It may not be sufficient to perfuse the vital organs.

Why should we care?

Patients in complete heart block may be asymptomatic depending upon ventricular escape mechanism and rate[25]. They may also present with symptoms ranging from lightheadedness to syncope and death. If you encounter this rhythm quickly assess your patient, anticipate the need for emergent external pacing, and notify the provider.

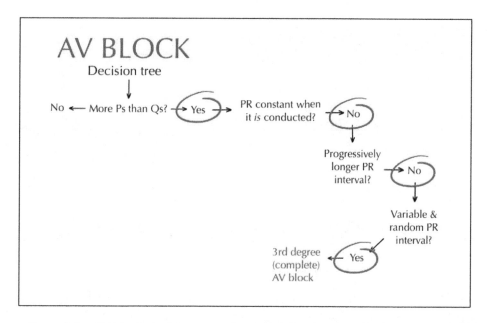

Review the portion of the AV block decision tree above that leads us to the determination of complete heart block.

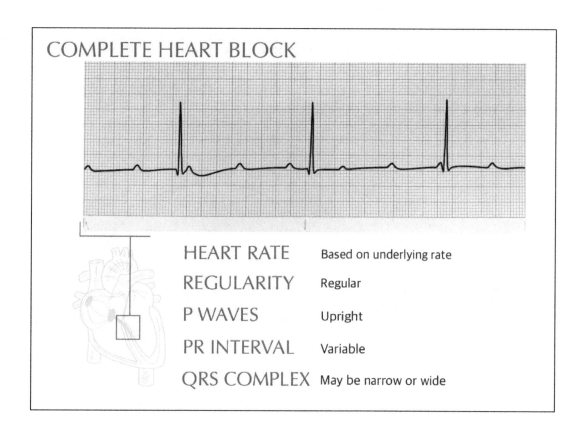

COMPLETE HEART BLOCK

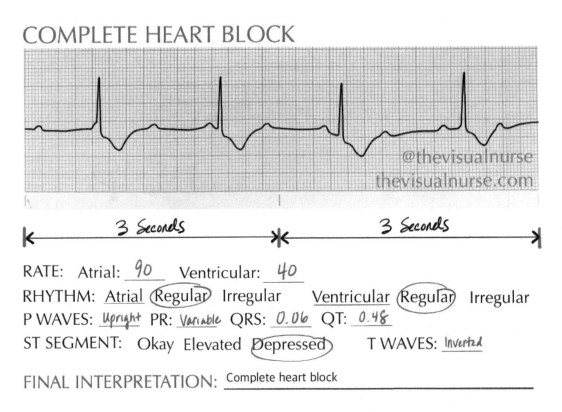

3 Seconds   3 Seconds

RATE: Atrial: _90_   Ventricular: _40_

RHYTHM: Atrial (Regular) Irregular   Ventricular (Regular) Irregular

P WAVES: _Upright_ PR: _Variable_ QRS: _0.06_ QT: _0.48_

ST SEGMENT: Okay Elevated (Depressed)   T WAVES: _Inverted_

FINAL INTERPRETATION: _Complete heart block_

Follow along with the sample rhythm interpretation above using the concepts that we've discussed to this point. Notice the constantly changing PR interval above. This is a hallmark finding of a complete heart block. This wraps up the cardiac rhythms and arrhythmias surrounding our inherent cardiac pacemaker cells. In our final section, we look at artificial pacemakers.

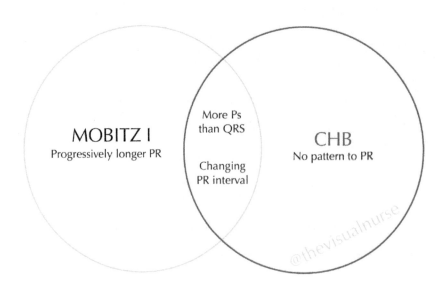

MOBITZ I
Progressively longer PR

More Ps than QRS

Changing PR interval

CHB
No pattern to PR

One final graphic on AV blocks. Never get fooled by these two again.

ATRIOVENTRICULAR BLOCK PRACTICE

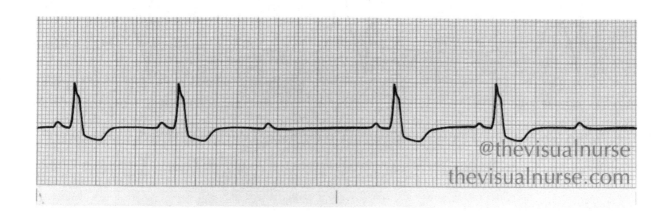

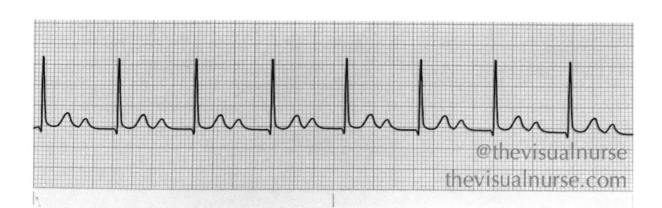

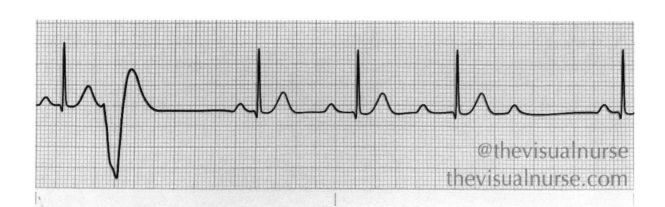

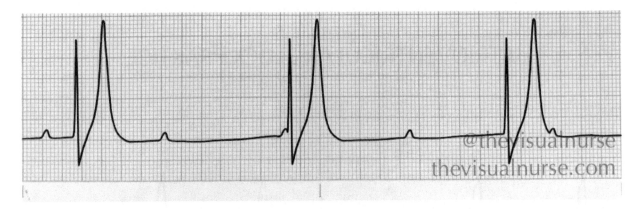

Turn to the "Rhythm strips answer key" section in the back of the book to check your answers!

CHAPTER 10: PACEMAKERS

ATRIAL
PACED

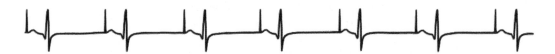

VENTRICULAR
PACED

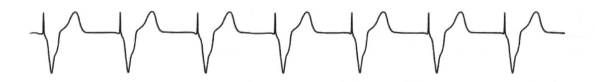

AV PACED

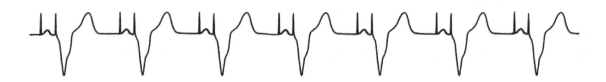

Overview of pacemaker therapy

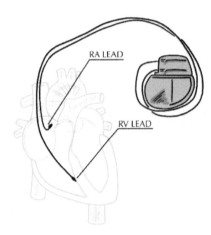

What are artificial pacemakers?

Natural pacemakers and artificial pacemakers exist. Natural pacemakers include the SA node and others downstream in the cardiac conduction system (i.e. atrial ectopics, junctional sites). Recall that the SA node is referred to as the "pacemaker of the heart" in many texts.

In some cases, the SA node might fail to generate an appropriate impulse (i.e. *sick sinus syndrome*). In contrast, the SA node may also generate an appropriate impulse that fails to result in ventricular activation (i.e. *complete heart block*). If any of these natural mechanisms fail, an artificial pacemaker may be needed to ensure ventricular stimulation and contraction in the presence of bradycardia.

What does this mean?

Artificial pacemakers stimulate depolarization and contraction similar to that of the cardiac pacemaker cells (namely the SA node). This stimulation shows up as a "pacemaker spike" on the ECG.

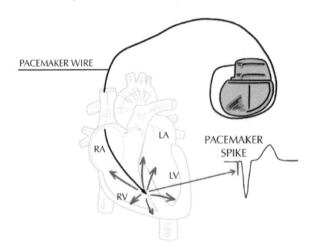

The goal with pacemaker therapy is to generate an impulse that stimulates depolarization and contraction at a rate that's sufficient to maintain appropriate cardiac output. Symptomatic bradycardia is the primary indication[35].

Pacemakers may be transcutaneous (defibrillator pads with pacemaker function), transvenous, or epicardial[17]; and either temporary or permanent. Permanent pacemakers are commonly single chamber or dual chamber[35]. Single chamber pacemakers possess a single pacemaker wire or lead placed in either the right atrium or right ventricle depending upon the indication. By comparison, dual chamber pacemakers possess two leads, one of which is typically placed in the right atrium and the other of which is placed in the right ventricle. Resynchronization devices may have a third lead placed in the left ventricle and newer devices may also pace directly into the bundle of His[35].

Capture: Ideally, each pacemaker spike results in a deflection that follows on the ECG. If a pacemaker spike is present with a deflection that follows, this indicates depolarization. The pacemaker is said to have *captured*.

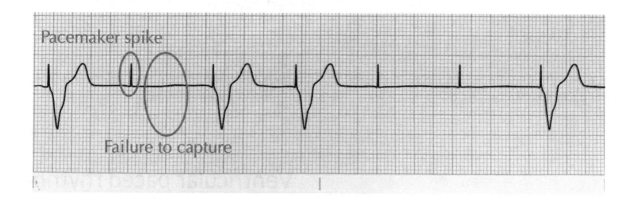

Capture is term that simply means the pacemaker signal resulted in depolarization of the cardiac tissue. If a pacemaker spike is present without a waveform following, the pacemaker is *failing to capture*[17] (above).

Atrial paced rhythms

ATRIAL PACED

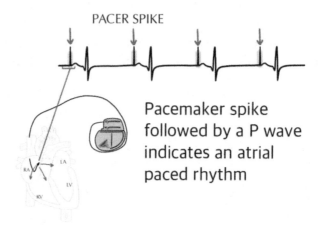

PACER SPIKE

Pacemaker spike
followed by a P wave
indicates an atrial
paced rhythm

The waveform that follows the pacemaker spike will tell you which chamber was stimulated to contract. If the pacemaker spike is followed by a P wave, the patient is *atrial paced*.

Ventricular paced rhythms

VENTRICULAR PACED

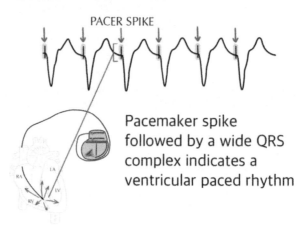

PACER SPIKE

Pacemaker spike
followed by a wide QRS
complex indicates a
ventricular paced rhythm

If the pacemaker spike is followed by a wide bizarre QRS complex the patient is *ventricular paced*.

Additionally, most pacemakers can "sense" intrinsic cardiac stimuli. In patients with a normal functioning SA node for example (i.e., with complete heart block), you may see a native P wave followed by a pacer spike, followed by a wide QRS. In these cases, the patient would be considered "*atrial sensed, ventricular paced*".

Atrioventricular paced rhythms

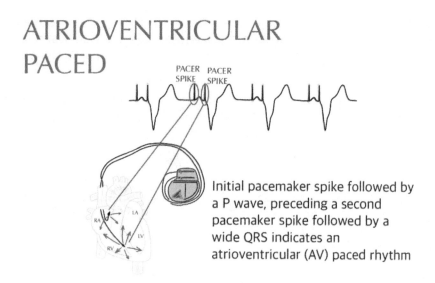

Initial pacemaker spike followed by a P wave, preceding a second pacemaker spike followed by a wide QRS indicates an atrioventricular (AV) paced rhythm

With two successive pacemaker spikes present; the first and second producing a P wave and a wide QRS, respectively, both the atria and ventricle are being artificially stimulated. These patients are *atrio-ventricular paced (AV paced)*.

Pacemakers are invaluable. They provide individuals with sometimes lethal conduction abnormalities the ability to live otherwise vibrant and healthy lives. Innovation through the years has increased quality of life as well as life expectancy for many grateful patients.

Why should we care?

Of course, technology is great if it's properly functioning. But pacemakers, just like any other device you may own has the potential to malfunction. For this reason, patients with permanent (implantable) pacemakers are scheduled for routine device checks in what is commonly referred to as the arrhythmia clinic, or device clinic.

Common malfunctions include:

- ✓ Failure to pace
- ✓ Failure to capture
- ✓ Failure to sense or under-sensing

Failure to pace

Failure to pace: this occurs when the pacemaker fails to deliver an appropriate impulse to stimulate myocardial depolarization, or it fails to reach the myocardium. This is recognized as a lack of pacemaker spikes where you would expect to see them. Expect to see a prolonged pause with no pacemaker activity. Causes may include oversensing, battery failure, and damaged or dislodged pacemaker leads[35].

Failure to capture

Failure to capture: we introduced this during our explanation of normal pacemaker functions. Capture is term that simply means the pacemaker signal resulted in depolarization of the cardiac tissue. If a pacemaker spike is present without a waveform following, the pacemaker is *failing to capture*, commonly a result of lead dislodgement, or increased thresholds for depolarization due to medications or electrolyte imbalances[35].

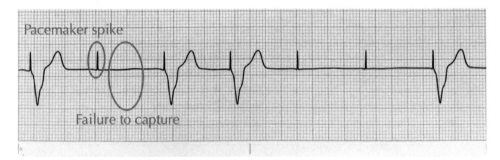

Failure to sense

Failure to sense; under-sensing: demand type pacemakers pace when they're needed. For example, if a patient has a permanent pacemaker due to profound symptomatic bradycardia that only occurs from time to time, they may have a *demand* pacemaker. If the patient can intrinsically pace on their own, the pacemaker should sense this and hold its activity. However, if the pacemaker fails to sense that the heart's native beats are adequately being produced and attempts to pace regardless of this, you'll see pacemaker spikes that occur inappropriately on the ECG strip. If the pacemaker is under-sensing, it over-paces. Expect to see pacemaker spikes in the middle of, or just after natural heart beats.

If you encounter any of the issues above, assess your patient. After you have ensured their stability and safety, notify the provider, and anticipate that the pacemaker representative will be called to perform a device interrogation for the purpose of uncovering the issue. Remember, pacemakers are stimulating the heart to depolarize. This means that just about any *natural* cause that would interfere with impulse transmission or mechanical contraction should be considered as a potential cause for malfunction.

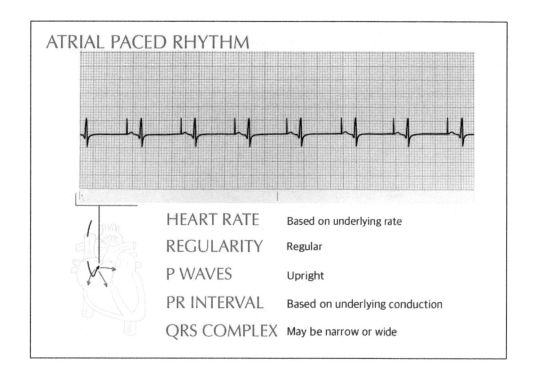

ATRIAL PACED RHYTHM

HEART RATE	Based on underlying rate
REGULARITY	Regular
P WAVES	Upright
PR INTERVAL	Based on underlying conduction
QRS COMPLEX	May be narrow or wide

ATRIAL PACED RHYTHM

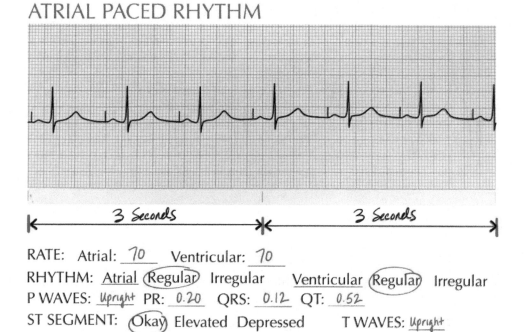

3 Seconds   3 Seconds

RATE: Atrial: _70_ Ventricular: _70_

RHYTHM: Atrial (Regular) Irregular   Ventricular (Regular) Irregular

P WAVES: Upright PR: _0.20_ QRS: _0.12_ QT: _0.52_

ST SEGMENT: (Okay) Elevated Depressed   T WAVES: Upright

FINAL INTERPRETATION: _Atrial paced rhythm_

Follow along with the sample rhythm interpretation above using the concepts that we've discussed to this point. Notice that each pacemaker spike is followed by a P wave, indicating that the atria are being artificially stimulated to depolarize.

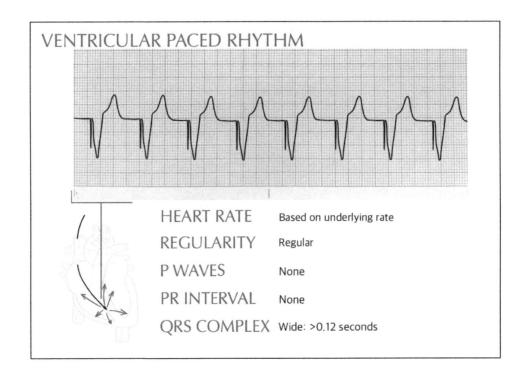

VENTRICULAR PACED RHYTHM

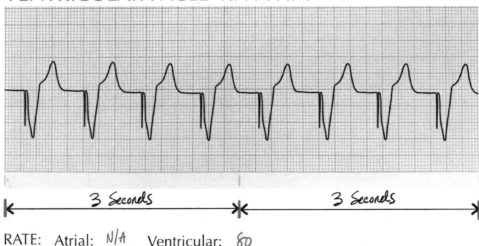

RATE: Atrial: _N/A_ Ventricular: _80_

RHYTHM: ~~Atrial~~ ~~Regular~~ ~~Irregular~~ Ventricular (Regular) Irregular

P WAVES: _N/A_ PR: _N/A_ QRS: _0.20_ QT: _0.48_

ST SEGMENT: Okay (Elevated) Depressed T WAVES: _Upright_

FINAL INTERPRETATION: ___Ventricular paced rhythm___

Follow along with the sample rhythm interpretation above using the concepts that we've discussed to this point. Notice that each pacemaker spike is followed by a wide and bizarre looking QRS complex, indicating that ventricles are being artificially stimulated to depolarize.

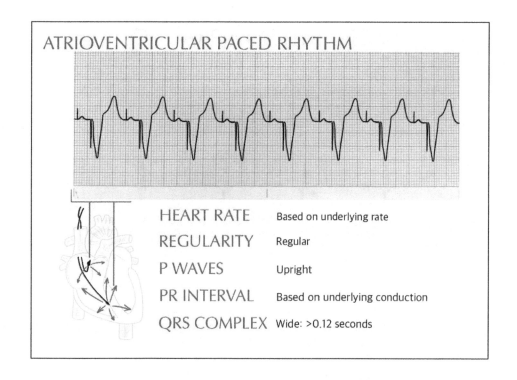

ATRIOVENTRICULAR PACED RHYTHM

HEART RATE	Based on underlying rate
REGULARITY	Regular
P WAVES	Upright
PR INTERVAL	Based on underlying conduction
QRS COMPLEX	Wide: >0.12 seconds

ATRIOVENTRICULAR PACED RHYTHM

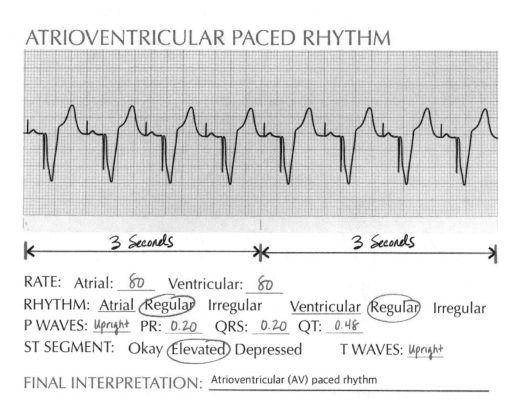

3 Seconds   3 Seconds

RATE: Atrial: _80_ Ventricular: _80_
RHYTHM: Atrial (Regular) Irregular   Ventricular (Regular) Irregular
P WAVES: Upright PR: _0.20_ QRS: _0.20_ QT: _0.48_
ST SEGMENT: Okay (Elevated) Depressed   T WAVES: Upright

FINAL INTERPRETATION: _Atrioventricular (AV) paced rhythm_

Follow along with the sample rhythm interpretation above using the concepts that we've discussed to this point. Notice that each initial pacemaker spike is followed by a P wave, which precedes a second pacemaker spike that's followed by a wide and bizarre looking QRS complex. This indicates that both the atria and ventricles are being artificially stimulated to depolarize.

PACED RHYTHM PRACTICE

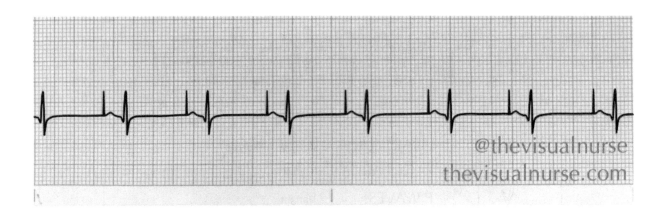

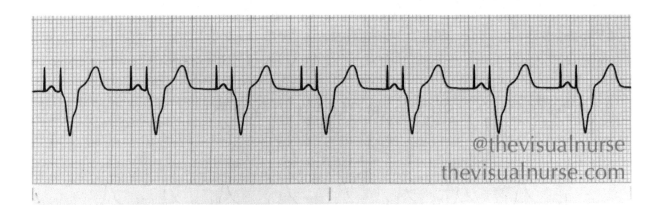

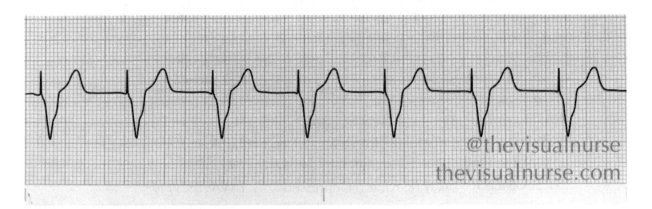

Turn to the "Rhythm strips answer key" section to check your answers!

INDEX OF RHYTHM PRACTICE ANSWER KEYS

SINUS ORIGIN PRACTICE STRIPS

Sinus rhythm with rate variation (Sinus arrhythmia)

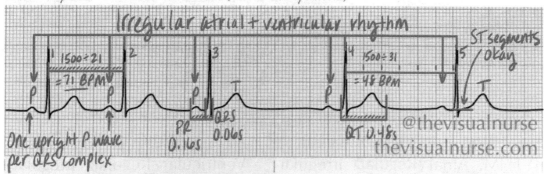

(6 second method)

RATE: Atrial: 50   Ventricular: 50

(Small box method)

Ventricular: 48-71 *

6 second method preferred for irregular rhythms

RHYTHM: Atrial Regular (Irregular)   Ventricular Regular (Irregular)

P WAVES: Upright PR: 0.16s QRS: 0.06s QT: 0.48s

ST SEGMENT: (Okay) Elevated Depressed   T WAVES: Upright

* In this example we can see why the 6 second method is preferred for rapid approximation

Sinus tachycardia w/ ST depression

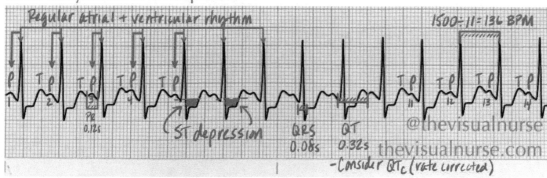

(6 second method)

RATE: Atrial: 140   Ventricular: 140

(Small box method)

Ventricular: 136

RHYTHM: Atrial (Regular) Irregular   Ventricular (Regular) Irregular

P WAVES: Upright PR: 0.12s QRS: 0.08s QT: 0.32s Consider QTc (rate)

ST SEGMENT: Okay Elevated (Depressed)   T WAVES: Upright

Sinus bradycardia with ST depression

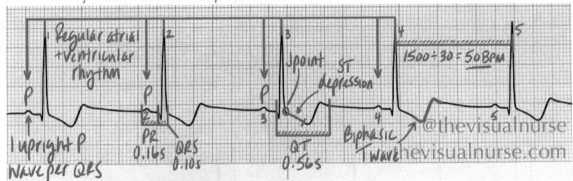

(6 second method) (Small box method)

RATE: Atrial: __50__ Ventricular: __50__ Ventricular: __50__

RHYTHM: Atrial (Regular) Irregular Ventricular (Regular) Irregular

P WAVES: Upright PR: 0.16s QRS: 0.10s QT: 0.56s

ST SEGMENT: Okay Elevated (Depressed) T WAVES: Biphasic

ATRIAL ORIGIN PRACTICE STRIPS

Uncontrolled atrial fibrillation

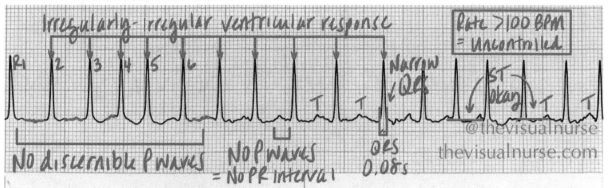

(6 second method)

RATE: ~~Atrial:~~ N/A Ventricular: 170   ~~Ventricular:~~

RHYTHM: ~~Atrial Regular Irregular~~ Ventricular Regular (Irregular)

P WAVES: N/A PR: N/A QRS: 0.08s QT: N/A or UTD

ST SEGMENT: (Okay) Elevated Depressed   T WAVES: Flat/upright

UTD: Unable to determine

Wandering atrial pacemaker

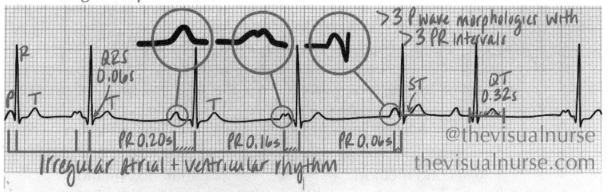

(6 second method)

RATE: Atrial: 70 Ventricular: 70   ~~Ventricular:~~

RHYTHM: Atrial Regular (Irregular) Ventricular Regular (Irregular)

P WAVES: Variable PR: Variable QRS: 0.06s QT: 0.32s

ST SEGMENT: (Okay) Elevated Depressed   T WAVES: Upright

Atrial flutter with 3:1 conduction

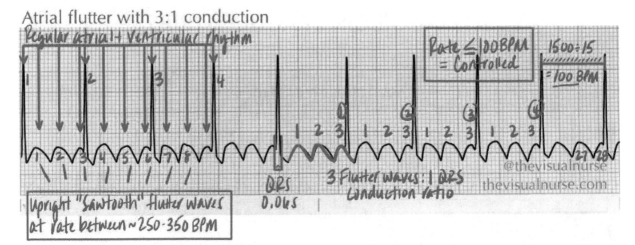

Regular atrial + ventricular rhythm

Rate ≤ 100 BPM = Controlled

1500 ÷ 15 = 100 BPM

QRS 0.04s

3 Flutter waves : 1 QRS conduction ratio

Upright "Sawtooth" flutter waves at rate between ~250-350 BPM

@thevisualnurse
thevisualnurse.com

	(6 second method)		(Small box method)

RATE: Atrial: 280   Ventricular: 100   Ventricular: 100

RHYTHM: Atrial (Regular) Irregular   Ventricular Regular (Irregular)

P WAVES: Upright PR: UTD   QRS: 0.04s QT: UTD

ST SEGMENT: ~~Okay Elevated Depressed~~ UTD   T WAVES: UTD

UTD - Unable to determine

Sinus rhythm with premature atrial contractions

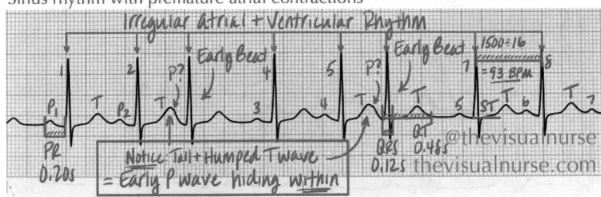

Irregular atrial + ventricular Rhythm

Early Beat

Early Beat

1500 ÷ 16 = 93 BPM

P₁   T   P₂   T   Early P wave   3   4   T   ST   5   6   T   7

PR 0.20s

Notice: Tall + Humped T wave = Early P wave hiding within

QRS 0.48s
0.12s

QT

@thevisualnurse
thevisualnurse.com

	(6 second method)		(Small box method)

RATE: Atrial: 70*   Ventricular: 80   Ventricular: 93*

RHYTHM: Atrial Regular (Irregular)   Ventricular Regular (Irregular)

P WAVES: Upright PR: 0.20s   QRS: 0.12s QT: 0.48s

ST SEGMENT: (Okay) Elevated Depressed   T WAVES: Upright

* Underlying rhythm, excluding early beats

JUNCTIONAL ORIGIN PRACTICE STRIPS

Junctional rhythm

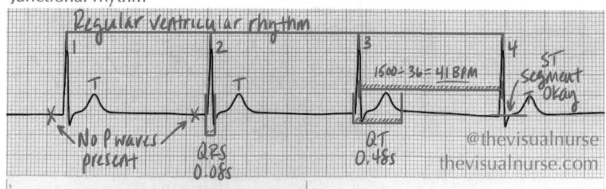

RATE: Atrial: N/A (6 second method) Ventricular: 40 (Small box method) Ventricular: 41

RHYTHM: ~~Atrial~~ ~~Regular~~ ~~Irregular~~ Ventricular (Regular) Irregular

P WAVES: N/A PR: N/A QRS: 0.08s QT: 0.48s

ST SEGMENT: (Okay) Elevated Depressed T WAVES: Upright

Supraventricular tachycardia with ST depression

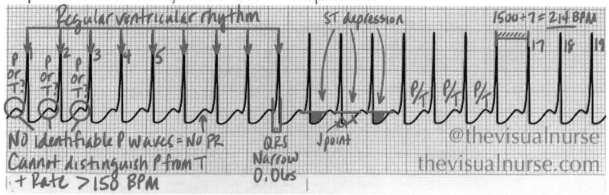

*No discernible P waves

RATE: Atrial: N/A (6 second method) Ventricular: 190 (Small box method) Ventricular: 214

RHYTHM: ~~Atrial~~ ~~Regular~~ ~~Irregular~~ Ventricular (Regular) Irregular

P WAVES: N/A PR: N/A QRS: 0.06s QT: N/A or UTD

ST SEGMENT: Okay Elevated (Depressed) T WAVES: N/A or upright

UTD - Unable to determine

Accelerated junctional rhythm

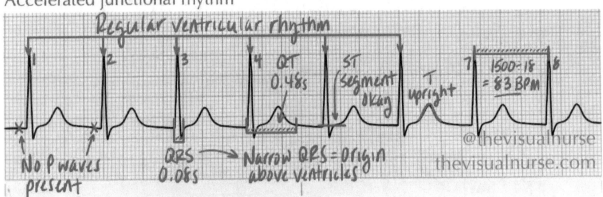

Regular ventricular rhythm

1   2   3   4 QT 0.48s   ST (segment okay)   T upright   7   1500÷18 = 83 BPM   8

No P waves present

QRS 0.08s → Narrow QRS = origin above ventricles

@thevisualnurse
thevisualnurse.com

	(6 second method)		(Small box method)

RATE: Atrial: N/A   Ventricular: 80   Ventricular: 83

RHYTHM: ~~Atrial~~ ~~Regular~~ ~~Irregular~~   Ventricular (Regular) Irregular

P WAVES: N/A   PR: N/A   QRS: 0.08s   QT: 0.48s

ST SEGMENT: (Okay) Elevated Depressed   T WAVES: Upright

VENTRICULAR ORIGIN PRACTICE STRIPS

Sinus/ sinus tachycardia with a run of non-sustained ventricular tachycardia (NSVT)

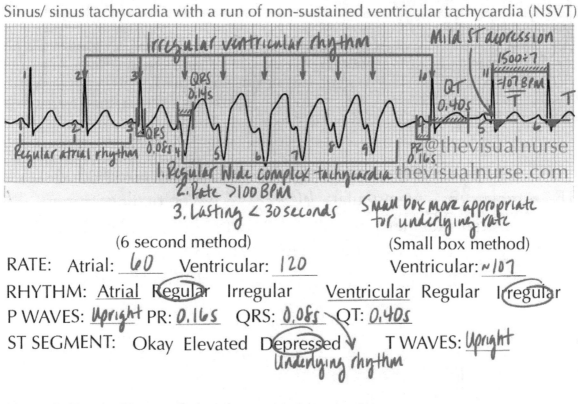

(6 second method)

RATE: Atrial: 60 Ventricular: 120   Ventricular: ~107 (Small box method)

RHYTHM: Atrial (Regular) Irregular   Ventricular Regular (Irregular)

P WAVES: Upright PR: 0.16s QRS: 0.08s QT: 0.40s

ST SEGMENT: Okay Elevated (Depressed) ↓   T WAVES: Upright

Sinus rhythm with a multifocal ventricular couplet

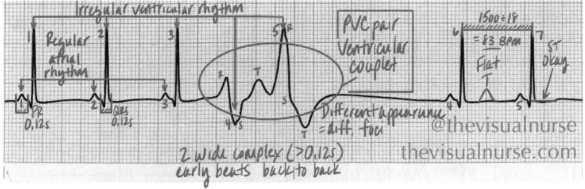

(6 second method)   Underlying rhythm (Small box method)

RATE: Atrial: 50 Ventricular: 70   Ventricular: 83

RHYTHM: Atrial (Regular) Irregular   Ventricular Regular (Irregular)

P WAVES: Upright PR: 0.12s QRS: 0.12s QT: Unable to determine

ST SEGMENT: (Okay) Elevated Depressed   T WAVES: Flat

Sinus bradycardia with a first degree AV delay, ventricular bigeminy and downsloping ST depression

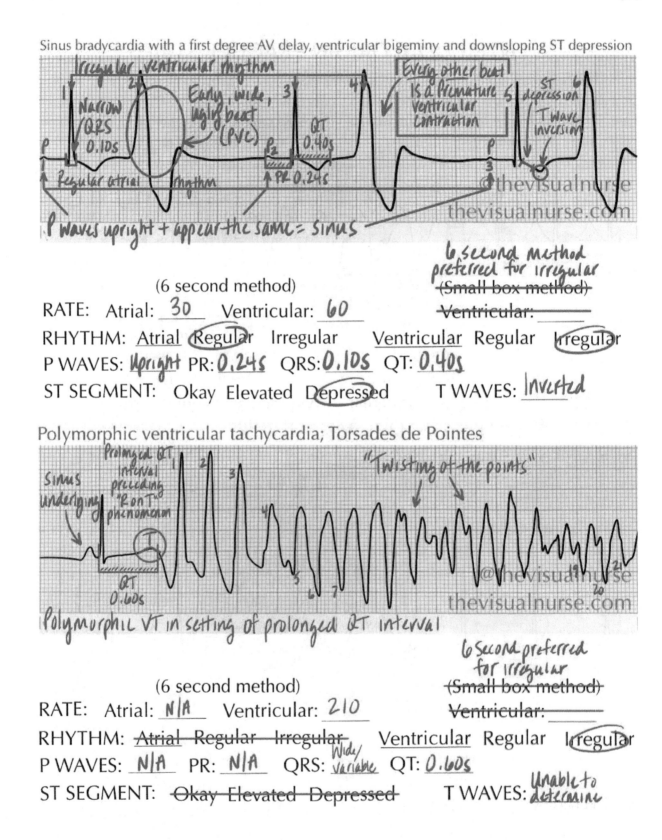

(6 second method)

RATE: Atrial: _30_ Ventricular: _60_ ~~Ventricular:~~ _____

RHYTHM: Atrial (Regular) Irregular Ventricular Regular (Irregular)

P WAVES: Upright PR: 0.24s QRS: 0.10s QT: 0.40s

ST SEGMENT: Okay Elevated (Depressed) T WAVES: Inverted

Polymorphic ventricular tachycardia; Torsades de Pointes

Polymorphic VT in setting of prolonged QT interval

(6 second method)

RATE: Atrial: _N/A_ Ventricular: _210_ ~~Ventricular:~~ _____

RHYTHM: ~~Atrial Regular Irregular~~ Ventricular Regular (Irregular)

P WAVES: _N/A_ PR: _N/A_ QRS: Wide/variable QT: 0.60s

ST SEGMENT: ~~Okay Elevated Depressed~~ T WAVES: Unable to determine

Accelerated idioventricular rhythm

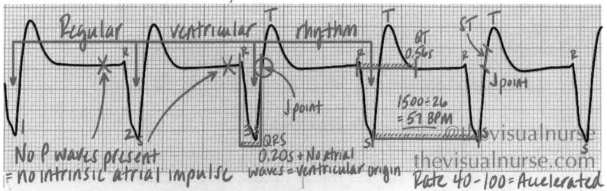

(6 second method)   (Small box method)

RATE: Atrial: __N/A__ Ventricular: __60__   Ventricular: __57__

RHYTHM: ~~Atrial Regular Irregular~~ Ventricular (Regular) Irregular

P WAVES: __N/A__ PR: __N/A__ QRS: __0.20s__ QT: __0.56s__

ST SEGMENT: Okay (Elevated) Depressed   T WAVES: Upright

Idioventricular rhythm

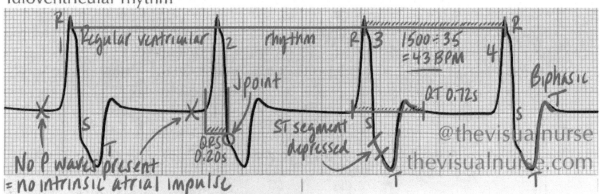

(6 second method)   (Small box method)

RATE: Atrial: __N/A__ Ventricular: __40__   Ventricular: __43__

RHYTHM: ~~Atrial Regular Irregular~~ Ventricular (Regular) Irregular

P WAVES: __N/A__ PR: __N/A__ QRS: __0.20s__ QT: __0.72s__ (Likely inaccurate)

ST SEGMENT: Okay Elevated (Depressed)   T WAVES: Biphasic

ATRIOVENTRICULAR BLOCK PRACTICE STRIPS

Sinus rhythm with second degree type II AV block; Mobitz II; with wide QRS & ST depression

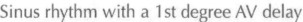

Irregular ventricular rhythm
Regular atrial rhythm
Wide QRS
Suspect underlying bundle block/ conduction delay
ST depression
QRS 0.16s
QT 0.48s
PR 0.16s
T
Consistent PR interval when conducted, with sporadic QRS drop
More P's than QRS
@thevisualnurse
thevisualnurse.com

6 second method preferred for irregular

(6 second method)

RATE: Atrial: 60   Ventricular: 40   ~~(Small box method)~~ ~~Ventricular:~~

RHYTHM: Atrial (Regular) Irregular   Ventricular Regular (Irregular)

P WAVES: Upright PR: 0.16s   QRS: 0.16s   QT: 0.48s

ST SEGMENT: Okay Elevated (Depressed)   T WAVES: Inverted

Sinus rhythm with a 1st degree AV delay

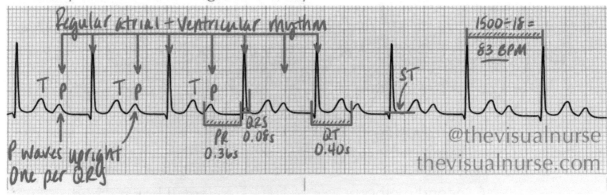

Regular atrial + ventricular rhythm
T P T P T P
ST
1500÷18 = 83 BPM
PR 0.36s   QRS 0.08s   QT 0.40s
P waves upright One per QRS
@thevisualnurse
thevisualnurse.com

(6 second method)   **(Small box method)**

RATE: Atrial: 80   Ventricular: 80   Ventricular: 83

RHYTHM: Atrial (Regular) Irregular   Ventricular (Regular) Irregular

P WAVES: upright PR: 0.36s   QRS: 0.08s   QT: 0.40s

ST SEGMENT: (Okay) Elevated Depressed   T WAVES: upright

Sinus rhythm with second degree type I AV block; Mobitz I; Wenckebach & isolated PVC

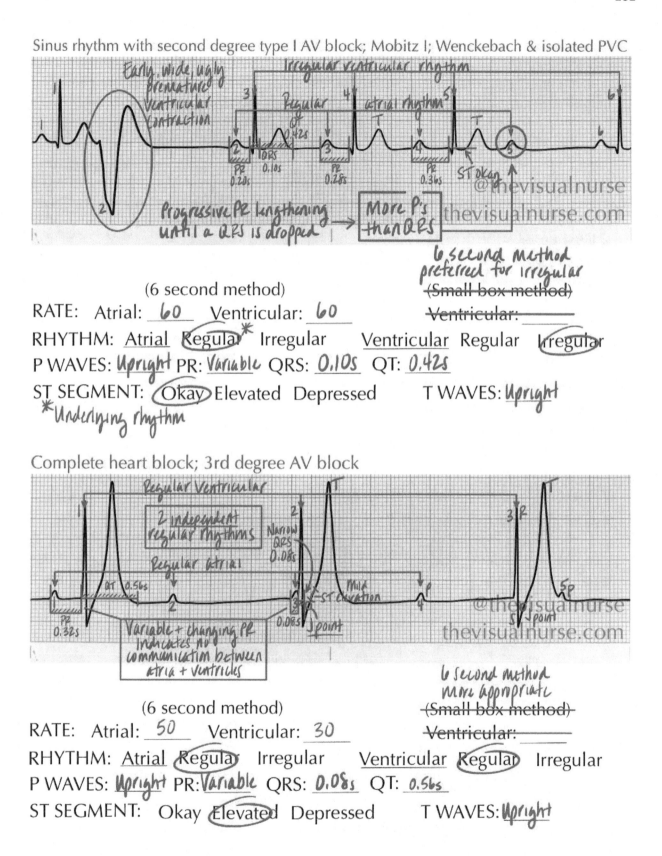

Early, wide, ugly Premature Ventricular Contraction

Irregular ventricular rhythm

Regular atrial rhythm

Progressive PR lengthening until a QRS is dropped →

More P's than QRS

6 second method preferred for irregular (Small box method)

(6 second method)

RATE: Atrial: 60   Ventricular: 60   ~~Ventricular:~~ _____

RHYTHM: Atrial (Regular)* Irregular   Ventricular Regular (Irregular)

P WAVES: Upright PR: Variable QRS: 0.10s QT: 0.42s

ST SEGMENT: (Okay) Elevated Depressed   T WAVES: Upright

*Underlying rhythm

Complete heart block; 3rd degree AV block

Regular Ventricular

2 independent regular rhythms

Narrow QRS 0.08s

Regular atrial

Variable + changing PR indicates no communication between atria + ventricles

Mild ST elevation   J point

ST ↓ point

6 second method more appropriate (Small box method)

(6 second method)

RATE: Atrial: 50   Ventricular: 30   ~~Ventricular:~~ _____

RHYTHM: Atrial (Regular) Irregular   Ventricular (Regular) Irregular

P WAVES: Upright PR: Variable QRS: 0.08s QT: 0.56s

ST SEGMENT: Okay (Elevated) Depressed   T WAVES: Upright

PACEMAKER PRACTICE STRIPS

Atrial paced rhythm

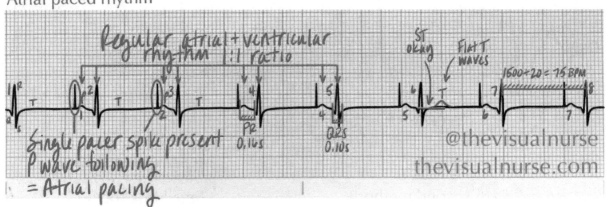

(6 second method)   (Small box method)

RATE: Atrial: _70_   Ventricular: _80_   Ventricular: _75_

RHYTHM: Atrial **Regular** Irregular   Ventricular **Regular** Irregular

P WAVES: Upright   PR: _0.16s_   QRS: _0.10s_   QT: Unable to determine

ST SEGMENT: **Okay** Elevated Depressed   T WAVES: _Flat_

Atrioventricular paced rhythm

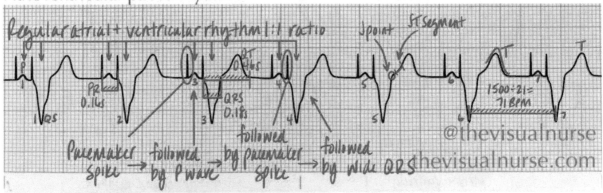

(6 second method)   (Small box method)

RATE: Atrial: _70_   Ventricular: _70_   Ventricular: _71_

RHYTHM: Atrial **Regular** Irregular   Ventricular **Regular** Irregular

P WAVES: Upright   PR: _0.16s_   QRS: _0.18s_   QT: _0.46s_

ST SEGMENT: Okay **Elevated** Depressed   T WAVES: _Upright_

Ventricular paced rhythm

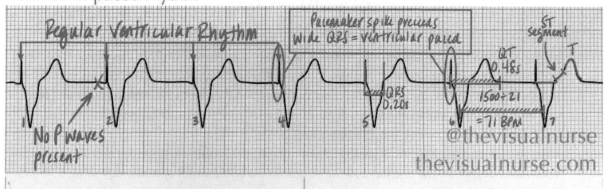

Regular Ventricular Rhythm

Pacemaker spike precedes wide QRS = ventricular paced

No P waves present

QRS 0.20s

1500÷21 = 71 BPM

QT 0.48s

ST segment

T

@thevisualnurse
thevisualnurse.com

(6 second method)

RATE: Atrial: N/A   Ventricular: 70

(Small box method)

Ventricular: 71

RHYTHM: ~~Atrial Regular Irregular~~   Ventricular (Regular) Irregular

P WAVES: N/A   PR: N/A   QRS: 0.20s   QT: 0.48s

ST SEGMENT: Okay (Elevated) Depressed   T WAVES: Upright

REFERENCES

1. Kligfield, P., Gettes, L.S., Bailey, J.J., Childers, R., Deal, B.J., Hancock, E.W., van Herpen, G., Kors, J.A., Macfarlane, P., Mirvis, D.M., Pahlm, O., Rautaharju, P., Wagner, G.S. (2007). Recommendations for the standardization and interpretation of the electrocardiogram: part I: The electrocardiogram and its technology. *Circulation, 115*(10), 1306-24. doi: 10.1161/CIRCULATIONAHA.106.180200.

2. Villa, A., Sammut, E., Nair, A., Rajani, R., Bonamini, R., & Chiribiri, A. (2016). Coronary artery anomalies overview: The normal and the abnormal. *World Journal of Radiology.* 8(6): 537-555. doi: 10.4329/wjr.v8.i6.537

3. Serrano, C. V., Jr, Bortolotto, L. A., César, L. A., Solimene, M. C., Mansur, A. P., Nicolau, J. C., & Ramires, J. A. (1999). Sinus bradycardia as a predictor of right coronary artery occlusion in patients with inferior myocardial infarction. *International journal of cardiology, 68*(1), 75–82. doi: 10.1016/s0167-5273(98)00344-1

4. Levin, D, B., & Perpetua, E. M. (2021). Cardiac anatomy and physiology. In E. M. Perpetua & P. A. Keegan (Eds.), *Cardiac nursing: The red reference book for cardiac nurses* (pp. 15-66). Wolters Kluwer.

5. Goldberger, J. J., Albert, C. M., & Myerburg, R. J. (2022). Cardiac arrest and sudden cardiac death. In P. Libey, R. O. Bonow, D. L. Mann, G. G. Tomaselli, D. L. Bhatt, S. D. Solomon, & E. Braunwald (Eds.) Heart disease: A textbook of cardiovascular medicine (pp. 1349-1386). Elsevier.

6. Cunningham, S.G., Brashers, V.L., & McCance, K.L. (2017). Structure and function of the cardiovascular and lymphatic systems. In V.L. Brashers & N.S. Rote (Eds.), *Understanding pathophysiology.* (pp. 569-597). Elsevier.

7. Kenney, W.,L., Wilmore J.H., & Costill, D.L. (2015). The cardiovascular system and its control. In A. N. Tocco, K. Maurer, K. Walsh, & J. Sexton (Eds.), *Physiology of sport and exercise.* (pp. 151-173). Human Kinetics.

8. Vincent J. L. (2008). Understanding cardiac output. *Critical care (London, England), 12*(4), 174. doi: 10.1186/cc6975

9. Bers, D. M., & Borlaug, B. A. (2022). Mechanisms of cardiac contraction and relaxation. In P. Libey, R. O. Bonow, D. L. Mann, G. G. Tomaselli, D. L. Bhatt, S. D. Solomon, & E. Braunwald (Eds.) Heart disease: A textbook of cardiovascular medicine (pp. 889-912). Elsevier.

10. Morrow, D. A., & De Lemos, J. (2022). Stable ischemic heart disease. In P. Libey, R. O. Bonow, D. L. Mann, G. G. Tomaselli, D. L. Bhatt, S. D. Solomon, & E. Braunwald (Eds.) Heart disease: A textbook of cardiovascular medicine (pp. 739-785). Elsevier.

11. Antzelevitch, C., & Burashnikov, A. (2011). Overview of Basic Mechanisms of Cardiac Arrhythmia. *Cardiac electrophysiology clinics, 3*(1), 23–45. doi: 10.1016/j.ccep.2010.10.012

12. Crossman D. C. (2004). The pathophysiology of myocardial ischaemia. *Heart (British Cardiac Society), 90*(5), 576–580. doi: 10.1136/hrt.2003.029017

13. Mirvis, D. M., & Goldberger, A. L. (2022). Electrocardiography. In P. Libey, R. O. Bonow, D. L. Mann, G. G. Tomaselli, D. L. Bhatt, S. D. Solomon, & E. Braunwald (Eds.) Heart disease: A textbook of cardiovascular medicine (pp. 141-174). Elsevier.

14. Nattel, S., & Tomaselli, G. F. (2022). Mechanisms of cardiac arrhythmias. In P. Libey, R. O. Bonow, D. L. Mann, G. G. Tomaselli, D. L. Bhatt, S. D. Solomon, & E. Braunwald (Eds.) Heart disease: A textbook of cardiovascular medicine (pp. 1163-1190). Elsevier.

15. Huether, S.E. (2017). Structure and function of the digestive system. In V.L. Brashers & N.S. Rote (Eds.), *Understanding pathophysiology*. (pp. 884-905). Elsevier.

16. Gildea, T. H., & Levis, J. T. (2018). ECG Diagnosis: Accelerated Idioventricular Rhythm. *The Permanente journal*, *22*, 17–173. doi: 10.7812/TPP/17-173

17. Mosely, M.J. (2021). Dysrhythmia interpretation and management. In M.L. Sole, D.G. Klein, M.J. Mosely, M.B. Flynn Makic, & M.T. Morata (Eds.), *Introduction to critical care nursing*. (pp. 105-145). Elsevier.

18. Stevenson, W. G., & Zeppenfeld, K. (2022). Ventricular arrhythmias. In P. Libey, R. O. Bonow, D. L. Mann, G. G. Tomaselli, D. L. Bhatt, S. D. Solomon, & E. Braunwald (Eds.) Heart disease: A textbook of cardiovascular medicine (pp. 1288-1311). Elsevier.

19. Katz, A. M. (2011). The electrocardiogram. In F. DeStefano (Ed.), Physiology of the heart. (pp. 401-430). Lippincott, Williams, & Wilkins.

20. Kalman, J. M., & Sanders, P. (2022). Supraventricular tachycardias. In P. Libey, R. O. Bonow, D. L. Mann, G. G. Tomaselli, D. L. Bhatt, S. D. Solomon, & E. Braunwald (Eds.) Heart disease: A textbook of cardiovascular medicine (pp. 1245-1271). Elsevier.

21. Holmqvist, F., & Daubert, J. P. (2013). First-degree AV block-an entirely benign finding or a potentially curable cause of cardiac disease? *Annals of noninvasive electrocardiology. 18*(3), 215–224. doi: 10.1111/anec.12062

22. Zheng, T. (2021). Electrocardiography and cardiac rhythm. In E. M. Perpetua & P. A. Keegan (Eds.), *Cardiac nursing: The red reference book for cardiac nurses* (pp. 289-359). Wolters Kluwer.

23. Balci B. (2009). Tombstoning ST-Elevation Myocardial Infarction. *Current cardiology reviews*, *5*(4), 273–278. doi: 10.2174/157340309789317869

24. Katz, A. M. (2011). Arrhythmias. In F. DeStefano (Ed.), Physiology of the heart. (pp. 432-487). Lippincott, Williams, & Wilkins.

25. Patton, K. K., Olgin, J. E. (2022). Bradyarrhythmias and atrioventricular block. In P. Libey, R. O. Bonow, D. L. Mann, G. G. Tomaselli, D. L. Bhatt, S. D. Solomon, & E. Braunwald (Eds.) Heart disease: A textbook of cardiovascular medicine (pp. 1312-1320). Elsevier.

26. Aburawi, E. H., Narchi, H., & Souid, A. K. (2013). Persistent wandering atrial pacemaker after epinephrine overdosing - a case report. *BMC pediatrics*, *13*, 1. doi: 10.1186/1471-2431-13-1

27. Calkins, H., Tomaselli, G. F., & Morady, F. (2022). Atrial fibrillation: Clinical features, mechanisms, and management. In P. Libey, R. O. Bonow, D. L. Mann, G. G. Tomaselli, D. L. Bhatt, S. D. Solomon, & E. Braunwald (Eds.) Heart disease: A textbook of cardiovascular medicine (pp. 1272-1287). Elsevier.

28. Markides, V., & Schilling, R. J. (2003). Atrial fibrillation: classification, pathophysiology, mechanisms and drug treatment. *Heart (British Cardiac Society)*, *89*(8), 939–943. doi: 10.1136/heart.89.8.939

29. Page, R. L., Joglar, J. A., Caldwell, M. A., Calkins, H., Conti, J. B., Deal, B. J., Estes, N. A., Field, M. E., Goldberger, Z. D., Hammill, S. C., Indik, J. H., Lindsay, B. D., Olshansky, B., Russo, A. M., Shen, W. K., Tracy, C. M., & Al-Khatib, S. M., (2016). 2015 ACC/AHA/HRS Guideline for the management of adult patients with supraventricular tachycardia: Executive summary: A report of the American College of Cardiology/American Heart Association Task Force on Clinical

Practice Guidelines and the Heart Rhythm Society. *Circulation*, *133*(14), e471–e505. doi: 10.1161/CIR.0000000000000310

30. Garner, J. B., & Miller, J. M. (2013). Wide Complex Tachycardia - Ventricular Tachycardia or Not Ventricular Tachycardia, That Remains the Question. *Arrhythmia & electrophysiology review*, *2*(1), 23–29. doi: **10.15420/aer.2013.2.1.23**

31. Giudicessi, J. R., Tester, D. J., & Ackerman, M., J. (2022). Genetics of cardiac arrhythmias. In P. Libey, R. O. Bonow, D. L. Mann, G. G. Tomaselli, D. L. Bhatt, S. D. Solomon, & E. Braunwald (Eds.) Heart disease: A textbook of cardiovascular medicine (pp. 1191-1207). Elsevier.

32. American Heart Association. (2020). *Adult cardiac arrest algorithm.* American Heart Association CPR and emergency cardiovascular care. https://cpr.heart.org/en/resuscitation-science/cpr-and-ecc-guidelines/algorithms

33. Gopinathannair, R., & Olshansky, B. (2009). Resting sinus heart rate and first degree av block: modifiable risk predictors or epiphenomena? *Indian pacing and electrophysiology journal*, *9*(6), 334–341.

34. Drew, B.J., Califf, R.M., Funk, M., Kaufman, E.S., Krucoff, M., Laks, M.M., Macfarlane, P.W., Sommargren, P., Swiryn, S., & Van Hare, G.F. (2004). Practice Standards for Electrocardiographic Monitoring in Hospital Settings. *Circulation*. *110*(17), 2721-2746. doi: 10.1161/01.CIR.0000145144.56673.59

35. Chung, M. K., & Daubert, J. P. (2022). Pacemakers and implantable cardioverter-defibrillators. In P. Libey, R. O. Bonow, D. L. Mann, G. G. Tomaselli, D. L. Bhatt, S. D. Solomon, & E. Braunwald (Eds.) Heart disease: A textbook of cardiovascular medicine (pp. 1321-1348). Elsevier.

INDEX

Made in the USA
Las Vegas, NV
17 December 2023

83088576R00109